Better Eyesight Without Glasses

Here is a book on eye-care and treatment which, soon after its first publication in 1919, came to be regarded as a classic. It is based on the author, Dr. W.H. Bates' own experiences in treating patients, and presents his theories which later on became normal practice everywhere.

The book is written in a simple and lucid style within easy grasp of the layreader. It discusses in detail the eye, its functioning, its diseases and their treatment, and also how to keep one's eyes normal and in healthy condition. He lays great stress on natural methods such as palming and central fixation (which is *tratak* in Indian parlance), and also on home treatment whenever needed. He proved once for all that good eyesight without glasses was not a myth but a reality within the reach of every person.

"...a worthwhile and inexpensive book and would certainly prove useful to those who follow the exercises given here."

Pioneer

BETTER EYESIGHT WITHOUT GLASSES

Dr. William H. Bates, M.D.

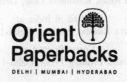

**Orient
Paperbacks**

DELHI | MUMBAI | HYDERABAD

ISBN 81-222-0021-4

1st Revised Orient Paperbacks edition 1984
17th Printing 2004

Better Eyesight Without Glasses

© Vision Books Pvt. Ltd.

Cover design by
C.V. Gurunathan for Vision Studio

Published by
Orient Paperbacks
(A division of Vision Books Pvt. Ltd.)
Madarsa Road, Kashmere Gate, Delhi-110 006

Printed in India at
Rashtra Rachna Printers, Delhi-110 092

Cover Printed at
Ravindra Printing Press, Delhi-110 006

TO THE MEMORY
OF THE
PIONEERS OF OPHTHALMOLOGY
THIS BOOK IS GRATEFULLY DEDICATED

I also gratefully acknowledge my indebtedness to Emily A. Bates, whose cooperation during four years of arduous labour and repeated failure made it possible to carry the work to a successful conclusion.

The Author

Dr. William H. Bates was born in Newark, New Jersey, in 1860, graduated from Cornell in 1881, received his medical degree from the College of Physicians and Surgeons in 1885. He established a practice in New York City, served for a time as clinical assistant at the Manhattan Eye and Ear Hospital, was attending physician at Bellevue Hospital in 1886-88, and at the New York Eye Infirmary, the Northern Dispensary and the Northeastern Dispensary in 1886-96. From 1886-91 he was an instructor in ophthalmology at the New York Postgraduate Medical School and Hospital. In 1896 Dr. Bates resigned his hospital appointments for several years of experimental work, returning to New York as attending physician in the Harlem Hospital from 1907-22. In 1919 he published the book of which this present volume is the revised edition. Never wholly in favour with the medical profession though with the highest medical training that his country could provide, his researches led him to the discovery of an entirely new theory of the eye's method of functioning. which has in turn led to a new trend in the treatment of defective eyesight, that has flourished in recent years.

Contents

Contents

1

The Theory and the Facts

MOST writers on ophthalmology appear to believe that the last word about problems of refraction (the deviation of light waves as they enter the eye) has been spoken, and according to their theories the last word is a very depressing one. Almost everyone in these days suffers from some form of refractive error. Yet we are told that for these ills, which not only are inconvenient but often are distressing and dangerous, there is no cure, no palliative except those optic crutches known as eyeglasses, and, under modern conditions of life, practically no preventive measure.

It is a well-known fact that the human body is not a perfect mechanism. Nature, in the evolution of the human tenement, has been guilty of some maladjustments. She has left behind, for instance, some troublesome bits of scaffolding, like the vermiform appendix. But nowhere is she supposed to have blundered so badly as in the construction of the eye. With one accord ophthalmologists tell us that the visual organ of man was never intended for the uses to which it is now put.

Eons before there were any schools or printing presses, electric lights or moving pictures, the evolution of the eye was complete. In those days it served the needs of the human animal perfectly. Man was a hunter, a herdsman, a farmer, a fighter. He needed, we are told, mainly distant vision; and since the eye at rest is adjusted for distant vision, sight is supposed to have been ordinarily as passive as the perception of sound, requiring no muscular action whatever. Near vision, it is assumed, was the exception, necessitating a muscular adjustment of such short duration that it was accomplished without placing any appreciable burden upon the mechanism of accommodation (the adjustment of the eye to different distances). The fact that primitive woman was a seamstress, an embroiderer, a weaver, an artist in all sorts of fine and beautiful work, appears to have been generally forgotten. Yet women living under primitive conditions have just as good eye-sight as the men.

When man learned how to communicate his thoughts to others by means of written and printed forms, there came some undeniably new demands upon the eye, affecting at first only a few people but gradually including more and more, until now, in the more advanced countries, the great mass of the population is subjected to their influence. A few hundred years ago even princes were not taught to read and write. Now we compel everyone to go to school, whether he wishes to or not, and even babies are sent to kindergarten. A generation or so ago books were scarce and expensive. Today, by means of libraries of all sorts, stationary and travelling, they have been brought within the reach of almost everyone. The modern newspaper, with its endless columns of badly printed reading matter, was made possible by the discovery of the art of manufacturing paper from wood, which is a thing of yesterday. Only lately has the tallow candle been displaced by the

10

various forms of artificial lighting, which tempt most of us to prolong our vocations and avocations into hours during which primitive man was forced to rest. Even more recently has come the moving picture to complete the supposedly destructive process.

Was it reasonable to expect that Nature should have provided for all these developments and produced an organ that could respond to the new demands? It is the accepted belief of ophthalmology today that she could not and did not, and that, while the processes of civilization depend upon the sense of sight more than upon any other, the visual organ is imperfectly fitted for its tasks.

There are a great number of facts which seem to justify this conclusion. While primitive man appears to have suffered little from defects of vision, it is safe to say that of persons over twenty-one living under civilized conditions, nine out of every ten have imperfect sight, and as the age increases the proportion increases, until at forty it is almost impossible to find a person free from visual defects. Voluminous statistics prove these assertions.

For more than a hundred years the medical profession has been seeking some method of checking the ravages of civilization upon the human eye. The Germans, to whom the matter has been one of vital military importance, have spent millions of dollars in carrying out the suggestions of experts, but without avail; and it is now admitted by most students of the subject that the methods which were once confidently advocated as reliable safeguards for the eye-sight of our children have accomplished little or nothing. Some take a more cheerful view of the matter, but their conclusions are hardly borne out by the facts.

For the prevailing method of treatment, by means of artificial lenses which compensate for the refractive error of the eye, very little was ever claimed except that these contrivances neutralized the effects of the various conditions for which they were prescribed, as a crutch enables a lame man to walk. It has also been believed that they sometimes checked the progress of these conditions; but every ophthalmologist now knows that their usefulness for this purpose, if any, is very limited. In the case of myopia (short-sightedness), as long ago as 1916 some ophthalmologists realized that glasses and all ordinary methods at our command 'are of but little avail' in preventing either an increase in the error of refraction or the development of the very serious complications with which it is often associated.

I have been studying the refraction of the human eye for more than thirty years, and my observations fully confirm these conclusions as to the uselessness of all the methods heretofore employed for the prevention and treatment of errors of refraction. I was very early led to suspect, however, that the problem was by no means an unsolvable one.

Every ophthalmologist of any experience knows that the theory of the incurability of errors of refraction does not fit the observed facts. Not infrequently such cases recover spontaneously, or change from one form to another. It has long been the custom either to ignore these troublesome facts or to explain them away, and fortunately for those who consider it necessary to bolster up the old theories at all costs, the role attributed to the lens of the eye in accommodation offers, in the majority of cases, a plausible method of explanation.

According to this theory, which most of us learned at school, the eye changes its focus for vision at different distances by altering the curvature of the lens; and in seeking an explanation for the inconstancy of the theoretically constant error of refraction, the theorists hit upon the very ingenious idea of attributing to the lens a capacity for changing its curvature not only for the purpose of normal accommodation but also to cover up or to produce accommodative errors. In hypermetropia (commonly but improperly called far-sightedness, although the patient with such a defect can see clearly neither at the distance nor at the near-point) the eyeball is too short from the front to the back, and all rays of light, both the convergent ones coming from near objects and the parallel ones coming from distant objects, are focused behind the retina instead of upon it. In myopia it is too long from the front to the back, and while the divergent rays from near objects come to a point upon the retina, the parallel ones from distant objects do not reach it.

Both of these conditions are supposed to be permanent, the one congenital, the other acquired. Thus when persons who at one time appear to have hypermetropia or myopia appear at other times not to have them, or to have them in lesser degrees, it is not permissible to suppose that there has been a change in the shape of the eyeball. Therefore, in the case of the disappearance or lessening of hypermetropia, we are asked to believe that the eye, in the act of vision, both at the near-point and at the distance, increases the curvature of the lens sufficiently to compensate, in whole or in part, for the flatness of the eyeball. In myopia, on the contrary, we are told that the eye actually goes out of its way to produce the condition, or

13

to make an existing condition worse. In their words, the so-called 'ciliary muscle', believed to control the shape of the lens, is credited with a capacity for getting into a more or less continuous state of contraction, thus keeping the lens continuously in a state of convexity which, according to the theory, it ought to assume only for vision at the nearpoint.

These curious performances may seem unnatural to the lay mind, but ophthalmologists believe the tendency to indulge in them to be so ingrained in the constitution of the organ of vision that, in the fitting of glasses, it is customary to instill atropine—the 'drops' with which everyone who has visited an oculist is familiar—into the eye, for the purpose of paralyzing the ciliary muscle and thus, by preventing any change of curvature in the lens, bringing out 'latent hypermetropia' and getting rid of 'apparent myopia'.

The interference of the lens, however, is believed to account for only moderate degrees of variation in errors of refraction, and that only during the earlier years of life. For the higher ones, or those that occur after forty-five years of age, when the lens is supposed to have lost its elasticity to a greater or lesser degree, no plausible explanation has ever been found.

The disappearance of astigmatism, or changes in its character, present an even more baffling problem. This condition is due in most cases to an unsymmetrical change in the curvature of the cornea, resulting in failure to bring the light rays to a focus at any point, and the eye is supposed to possess only a limited ability to overcome it—and yet astigmatism comes and goes with as much facility as other errors of refraction. It is well known, too, that it can be produced voluntarily. Some persons can produce as much as three diopters

14

(a diopter is the focusing power necessary to bring parallel rays to a focus at one meter, or 39.37 inches). I myself can produce one and a half.

Examining thousands of pairs of eyes a year at the New York Eye and Ear Infirmary and other institutions I observed many cases in which errors of refraction either recovered spontaneously or changed their form, and I was unable either to ignore them or to satisfy myself with the orthodox explanations, even where such explanations were available. It seemed to me that if a statement is a truth it must always be a truth. There can be no exceptions. If errors of refraction are incurable, they should not recover, or change their form, spontaneously.

In the course of time I discovered that myopia and hypermetropia, like astigmatism, could be produced at will; that myopia was not, as we have so long believed, associated with the use of the eyes at the near-point, but with a strain to see distant objects, strain at the near-point being associated with hypermetropia; that no error of refraction was ever a constant condition; and that the lower degrees of refractive error could be eliminated, while higher degrees could be improved.

In seeking light upon these problems I examined tens of thousands of eyes, and the more facts I accumulated, the more difficult it became to reconcile them with the accepted views. Finally I undertook a series of observations upon the eyes of human beings and the lower animals, the results of which convinced both myself and others that the lens is not a factor in accommodation and that the adjustment necessary for vision at different distances is affected in the eye, precisely as it is in the camera, by a change in the length of the organ, this alteration being brought about by the action of the muscles on the outside of the eyeball. Equally convincing was the demonstration that errors of refraction, including presbyopia (rigidity of the lens, causing difficulty in accommodation and recession of the nearpoint), are due not to an organic change in the shape of the eyeball or in the constitution of the lens, but to a functional derangement in the action of the muscles on the outside of the eyeball, and therefore can be eliminated.

In making these statements I am well aware that I am controverting the practically undisputed teaching of ophthalmological science for the better part of a century, but I have been driven to my conclusions by the facts, and so slowly that I am now surprised at my own hesitation. At the time I was improving high degrees of myopia, but I wanted to be conservative and I differentiated between functional myopia, which I was able to eliminate or improve, and organic myopia, which, in deference to the orthodox tradition, for a time I accepted as incorrigible.

2

Simultaneous Retinoscopy

MUCH of my information about the eyes has been obtained by means of simultaneous retinoscopy—that is, clinical examination of the retina. The retinoscope is an instrument used to measure the refraction of the eye. It throws a beam of light into the pupil by reflection from a mirror, the light being either outside the instrument—above and behind the subject—or arranged within it by means of an electric battery. On looking through the sight-hole, one sees a larger or smaller part of the pupil filled with light, which in normal human eyes is a reddish yellow because this is the color of the retina. Unless the eye is exactly focused at the point from which it is being observed, one sees also a dark shadow at the edge of the pupil, and it is the behaviour of this shadow when the mirror is moved in various directions that reveals the refractive condition of the eye.

If the instrument is used at a distance of six feet or more and the shadow moves in a direction opposite to the movement of the mirror, the eye is myopic. If the shadow moves in the same direction as the mirror, the eye is either hypermetropic or normal; in the case of hypermetropia, the movement is more pronounced than in that of normality, and an expert can usually tell the

17

difference between the two states merely by the nature of the movement. In astigmatism the movement is different in different meridians. (A meridian is a vertical plane projected forward from the poles of the eyeball). To determine the degree of the error, or to distinguish accurately between hypermetropia and normality, or between the different kinds of astigmatism, it is usually necessary to experiment with a lens before the eye of the subject. If the mirror is concave instead of plane, the movements described will be reversed; the plane mirror is the one most commonly used, however.

The Snellen* test card and trial lenses can be used only under certain favourable conditions, but the retinoscope can be used anywhere. It is a little easier to use it in a dim light than in a bright one, but it may be used in any light, even with the strong light of the sun shining directly into the eye. It may also be used under many other unfavorable conditions.

It takes a considerable time, varying from minutes to hours, to measure the refraction with the Snellen test card and trial lenses. With the retinoscope, however, it can be determined in a fraction of a second. By the former method it would be impossible, for instance, to get any information about the refraction of a baseball player at the moment he swings for the ball, at the moment he strikes it, and at the moment after he strikes

*Herman Snellen (1835-1908), celebrated Dutch ophthalmologist, professor of ophthalmology at the University of Utrecht and director of the Netherlandic Eye Hospital. The present standards of visual acuity were proposed by him, and his test types became the model for those now in use. The test card is a chart by wh ch a person's visual power is measured.

18

it. But with the retinoscope it is quite easy to determine whether his vision is normal, or whether he is myopic, hypermetropic, or astigmatic, when he does these things; and if any errors of refraction are noted, one can guess their degree pretty accurately by the rapidity of the movement of the shadow.

With the test card and trial lenses conclusions must be drawn from the patient's statements as to what he sees. But the patient often becomes so worried and confused during the examination that he does not know what he sees, or whether different glasses make his sight better or worse; and, moreover, visual acuity is not reliable evidence of the refraction. One patient with two diopters of myopia may see twice as much as another with the same error of refraction. The evidence of the test card is, in fact, entirely subjective, while that of the retinoscope is entirely objective, depending in no way upon the statements of the patient.

In short, while the testing of the refraction by means of the test card and trial lenses requires considerable time, and can be done only under certain artificial conditions, with results that are not always reliable, the retinoscope can be used under all sorts of normal and abnormal conditions on the eyes of both human beings and the lower animals, and the results, when it is used properly, can always be depended upon. This means that it must not be brought nearer to the eye than six feet; otherwise the subject will be made nervous, and the refraction, for reasons which will be explained later, will be changed and no reliable observations will be possible. In the case of animals it is often necessary to use it at a much greater distance.

For thirty years I have been using the retinoscope to study the refraction of the eye. With it I have examined the eyes of tens of thousands of school children, hundreds of infants and thousands of animals, including cats, dogs, rabbits, horses, cows, birds turtles reptiles and fish. I have used it when the subjects were at rest and when they were in motion—also when I myself was in motion—when they were awake and when they were asleep or even under ether or chloroform. I have used it in the daytime and at night, when the subjects were comfortable and when they were excited; when they were trying to see and when they were not; when they were lying and when they were telling the truth; when the eyelids were partly closed, shutting off part of the area of the pupil; when the pupil was dilated and also when it was contracted to a pinpoint; when the eye was oscillating from side to side, from above downward and in other directions.

In this way I discovered many facts which had not previously been known, and which I was quite unable to reconcile with the orthodox teachings on the subject. This led me to undertake the series of experiments already alluded to. The results were in entire harmony with my previous observations, and left me no choice but to reject the entire body of orthodox teaching about accommodation and errors of refraction.

20

3

The Truth about Accommodation

THE testimony of my experiments proved to me that the lens is not a factor in accommodation. This fact is confirmed by numerous observations on the eyes of adults and children with normal vision, errors of refraction, or amblyopia (a decline of vision with no apparent cause), and on the eyes of adults after the removal of the lens for cataract.

It has already been pointed out that the instillation of atropine into the eye is supposed to prevent accommodation by paralyzing the muscle credited with controlling the shape of the lens. That it has this effect is generally accepted in every textbook on the subject, and the drug is used daily in the fitting of glasses for the purpose of eliminating the supposed influence of the lens upon refractive states.

In about nine cases out of ten the conditions resulting from the instillation of atropine into the eye fit the theory upon which its use is based, but in the tenth case they do not, and every ophthalmologist of any experience has noted some of these tenth cases. Many of them are reported in the literature of the subject; and many of them have come under my own observation. According to the theory, atropine ought to bring out latent hypermetropia in eyes either apparently normal

21

or manifestly hypermetropic, provided, of course, the patient is of the age during which the lens is supposed to retain its elasticity. The fact is, however, that it sometimes produces myopia or changes hypermetropia into myopia, and that it will produce both myopia and hypermetropia in persons over seventy years of age, when the lens is supposed to be as hard as a stone, as well as in cases in which the lens is hard with incipient cataract. Patients with apparently normal eyes, will after the use of atropine, develop hypermetropic astigmatism, or myopic astigmatism, or compound myopic astigmatism, or mixed astigmatism. In other cases the drug will not interfere with the accommodation or alter the refraction in any way. Furthermore, when the vision has been lowered by atropine the subjects have often become able, simply by resting their eyes, to read diamond type (the smallest type face commonly in use, now usually known as fine-print type—see illustration in Chapter 14 for an example) at six inches. Yet atropine is supposed to rest the eyes by affording relief to an overworked muscle.

In the treatment of squint and amblyopia I have often used atropine in the better eye for more than a year, in order to encourage the use of the amblyopic eye; and at the end of this time; while still under the influence of atropine, such eyes have become able, in a few hours or less, to read diamond type at six inches. The following are examples of many similar cases that might be cited.

A boy of ten had hypermetropia in both eyes, that of the left or better eye amounting to three diopters. When atropine was instilled into this eye, the hypermetropia was increased to four and a half diopters and the vision lowered to 20/200 (200/200 is normal; the num-

22

erator of the fraction is the distance at which the patient can see a letter on a test card, and the denominator is the distance at which he should be able to see it). With a convex glass of four and a half diopters the patient obtained normal vision for the distance, and with the addition of another convex glass of four diopters he was able to read diamond type at ten inches (best). The atropine was used for a year, the pupil being dilated continually to the maximum. Meantime the right eye was being treated by my own methods, which will be described later. Usually in such cases the eye which is not being specifically treated improves to some extent with the other, but in this case it did not. At the end of the year the vision of the right eye had become normal; but that of the left eye remained precisely what it was at the beginning, being still 20 200 without glasses for the distance, while reading without glasses was impossible and the degree of the hypermetropia had not changed. Still under the influence of the atropine and still with the pupil dilated to the maximum, this eye was now treated separately, and in half an hour its vision had become normal for both the distance and the near-point, diamond type being read at six inches, all without glasses. According to the accepted theories, the ciliary muscle of this eye must have been not only completely paralyzed at the time but in a state of complete paralysis for a year. Yet the eye not only overcame four and a half diopters of hypermetropia but added six diopters of accommodation, making a total of ten and a half. It remains for those who adhere to the accepted theories to say how such facts can be reconciled with them.

Equally if not more remarkable was the case of a little girl of six who had two and a half diopters of hypermetropia in her right or better eye, and six in the other with one diopter of astigmatism. With the better eye under the influence of atropine and the pupil dilated to the maximum, both eyes were treated together for more than a year, and at the end of that time, the right being still under the influence of the atropine, both became able to read diamond type at six inches, the right doing it better, if anything, than the left. Thus, in spite of the atropine, the right eye not only overcame two and a half diopters of hypermetropia but added six diopters of accommodation, making a total of eight and a half. In order to eliminate all possibility of latent hypermetropia in the left eye—which in the beginning had six diopters—the atropine was now used in this eye and discontinued in the other, the eye education being continued as before. Under the influence of the drug there was a slight return of the hypermetropia; but the vision quickly became normal again and although the atropine was used daily for more than a year, the pupil being continually dilated to the maximum, diamond type was read at six inches without glasses during the whole period. It is difficult for me to to see how the ciliary muscle could have had anything to do with the ability of this patient to accommodate after atropine had been used in each eye separately for a year or more at a time.

According to the current theory, as I have said, atropine paralyzes the ciliary muscle and thus, by preventing a change of curvature in the lens, prevents accommodation. When accommodation occurs, therefore, after the prolonged use of atropine, it is evident that it must be due to some factor or factors other than the lens and the ciliary muscle. The evidence of such cases against the accepted theories is, in fact, overwhel-

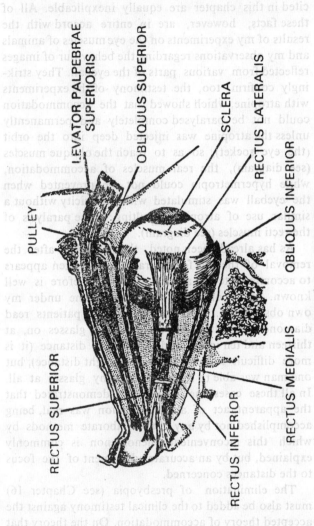

The Muscles of the Eye

ming, and according to these theories the other factors cited in this chapter are equally inexplicable. All of these facts, however, are in entire accord with the results of my experiments on the eye muscles of animals and my observations regarding the behaviour of images reflected from various parts of the eyeball. They strikingly confirm, too, the testimony of the experiments with atropine, which showed that the accommodation could not be paralysed completely and permanently unless the atropine was injected deep into the orbit (the eye socket), so as to reach the oblique muscles (see diagram), the real muscles of accommodation, while hypermetropia could not be prevented when the eyeball was stimulated with electricity without a similar use of atropine, resulting in the paralysis of the recti muscles (see diagram).

As has already been noted, the fact that after the removal of the lens for cataract the eye often appears to accommodate just as well as it did before is well known. Many of these cases have come under my own observation. Not only have such patients read diamond type with only their distance glasses on, at thirteen and ten inches and at a smaller distance (it is more difficult to read at a very slight distance), but one man was able to read without any glasses at all. In all these cases the retinoscope demonstrated that the apparent act of accommodation was real, being accomplished not by any of the elaborate methods by which this inconvenient phenomenon is commonly explained, but by an accurate adjustment of the focus to the distances concerned.

The elimination of presbyopia (see Chapter 16) must also be added to the clinical testimony against the accepted theory of accommodation. On the theory that the lens is a factor in accommodation, such a change would be manifestly impossible. The fact that rest for the eyes improves the sight in presbyopia has been noted by others and has been attributed to the supposed fact that the rested ciliary muscle is able for a brief period to influence the hardened lens; but while it is conceivable that this might happen in the early stages of the condition and for a few moments, it is not conceivable that permanent relief should be obtained by this means, or that lenses which are as the saying goes, as 'hard as stone' should be influenced even momentarily.

A truth is strengthened by an accumulation of facts. A working hypothesis is proved not to be a truth if a single fact is not in harmony with it. The accepted theories of accommodation and of the cause of errors of refraction require that a multitude of facts should be explained away. During more than thirty years of clinical experience, I have not observed a single fact that was not in harmony with the belief that the lens and the ciliary muscle have nothing to do with accommodation and that the changes in the shape of the eyeball upon which errors of refraction depend are not permanent. My clinical observations have of themselves been sufficient to demonstrate the truth of this belief. They have also been sufficient to show how errors of refraction can be produced at will, and how they may be eliminated temporarily in a few minutes and permanently by continued treatment.

4

The Variability of Refraction

THE theory that errors of refraction are due to permanent deformations of the eyeball leads naturally to the conclusion that errors of refraction are permanent states and that normal refraction is a continuous condition. As this theory is almost universally accepted as a fact, therefore, it is not surprising to find that the normal eye is generally regarded as a perfect machine which is always in good working order. No matter whether the object regarded is strange or familiar, whether the light is good or imperfect, whether the surroundings are pleasant or disagreeable, even under conditions of nerve strain or bodily disease, the normal eye is expected to have normal refraction and normal sight all the time. It is true that the facts do not harmonize with this view, but they are conveniently attributed to the perversity of the ciliary muscle, or, if that explanation will not work, ignored altogether.

When we understand, however, how the shape of the eyeball is controlled by the external muscles, and how it responds instantaneously to their action, it is easy to see that no refractive state, whether it is normal or abnormal, can be permanent. This conclusion is confirmed by the retinoscope, and I had observed the facts long before the experiments mentioned in the preceding chapters offered a satisfactory explanation for it. During thirty years devoted to the study of refraction, I have found few people who could maintain perfect sight—that is, with no refractive error—for more than a few minutes at a time, even under the most favourable conditions; and often I have seen the refraction change half a dozen times or more in a second, the variations ranging all the way from twenty diopters of myopia to normal.

Similarly, I have found no eyes with continuous or unchanging errors of refraction, all persons with errors of refraction having, at frequent intervals during the day and night, moments of normal vision when their myopia, hypermetropia, or astigmatism wholly disappears. The form of the error also changes, myopia even changing into hypermetropia and one form of astigmatism into another.

Of several thousand school children examined in one year, more than half had normal eyes, with sight which was perfect at times, but not one of them had perfect sight in each eye at all times of the day. Their sight might be good in the morning and imperfect in the afternoon, or imperfect in the morning and perfect in the afternoon. Many children could read one test card with perfect sight but were unable to see a different one perfectly. Many could also read some letters of the alphabet perfectly, while unable to distinguish other letters of the same size under similar conditions. The degree of this imperfect sight varied within wide limits, from one-third to one-tenth, or less. Its duration was also variable. Under some conditions it might continue for only a few minutes, or less; under others it might prevent the subject from seeing the blackboard for days, weeks, or even longer. Frequently all the pupils in a classroom were affected to this extent.

Among babies a similar condition was noted. Most investigators have found babies hypermetropic. A few have found them myopic. My own observations indicate that the refraction of infants is continually changing. One child was examined under atropine on four successive days, beginning two hours after birth. A three per cent solution of atropine was instilled into both eyes, the pupil was dilated to the maximum, and other physiological symptoms of the use of atropine were noted. The first examination showed a condition of mixed astigmatism. On the second day there was compound hypermetropic astigmatism, and on the third compound myopic astigmatism. On the fourth one eye was normal and the other showed simple myopia. Similar variations were noted in many other cases.

What is true of children and infants is equally true of adults of all ages. Persons over seventy years of age have suffered losses of vision of variable degree and intensity, and in such cases the retinoscope always indicated an error of refraction. A man eighty years old with normal eyes and ordinarily normal sight had periods of imperfect sight which would last from a few minutes to half an hour or longer. Retinoscopy at such times always indicated myopia of four diopters or more.

During sleep the refractive condition of the eye is rarely, if ever, normal. Persons whose refraction is normal when they are awake will produce myopia, hypermetropia and astigmatism when they are asleep. Or, if they have errors of refraction when they are awake, these will be increased during sleep. This is why

30

people awake in the morning with eyes more tired than at any other time, or even with severe headaches. When the subject is under ether or chloroform or is unconscious from any other cause, errors of refraction are also produced or increased.

When the eye regards an unfamiliar object, an error of refraction is always produced. Hence the proverbial fatigue caused by viewing pictures, or other objects, in a museum. Children with normal eyes who can read perfectly small letters a quarter of an inch high at ten feet always have trouble in reading strange writing on the blackboard, although the letters may be two inches high. A strange map, or any map, has the same effect. I have never seen a child, or a teacher, who could look at a map at a distance without becoming near-sighted. German type has been accused of being responsible for much of the poor sight once supposed to be peculiarly a German malady, but if a German child attempts to read Roman print he will at once become temporarily hypermetropic. German print, or Greek or Chinese characters, will have the same effect on a child, or other person, accustomed to Roman letters. Professor Hermann Cohn, of Breslau, repudiated the idea that German lettering was trying to the eyes. On the contrary, he always found it 'pleasant, after a long reading of the monotonous Roman print, to return "to our beloved German". Because the German characters were more familiar to him than any others he found them restful to his eyes. 'Use,' as he truly observed, 'has much to do with the matter.' Children learning to read, write, draw or sew always suffer from defective vision, because of the unfamiliarity of the lines or objects with which they are working.

31

A sudden exposure to strong light, or a rapid or sudden change of light, is likely to produce imperfect sight in the normal eye, continuing in some cases for weeks and months (see Chapter 16).

Noise is also a frequent cause of defective vision in the normal eye. All persons see imperfectly when they hear an unexpected loud noise. Familiar sounds do not lower the vision, but unfamiliar ones always do. Country children from quiet schools may suffer from defective vision for a long time after moving to a noisy city. In school they cannot do well with their work, because their sight is impaired. It is, of course, a gross injustice for teachers and others to scold, punish or humiliate such children.

Under conditions of mental or physical discomfort, such as pain, cough, fever, discomfort from heat or cold, depression, anger, or anxiety, errors of refraction are always produced in the normal eye or increased in the eye in which they already exist.

The variability of the refraction of the eye is responsible for many otherwise unaccountable accidents. When people are struck down in the street by automobiles or trolley cars, it is often because they are suffering from temporary loss of sight. Collisions on railroads or at sea, disasters in military operations, aviation accidents, etc., often occur because some responsible person suffered temporary loss of sight.

To this cause must also be ascribed, in a large degree, the confusion which every student of the subject has noted in the statistics which have been collected regarding the occurrence of errors of refraction. So far as I am aware, it has never been taken into account by any investigator of the subject, yet the result in any such investigation must be largely determined by the conditions under which it is made. It is possible to take the best eyes in the world and test them so that the subject will not be able to get into the Army. Again, the test may be so made that eyes which are apparently much below normal at the beginning may in the few minutes required for the test acquire normal vision and become able to read the test card perfectly.

5

What Glasses Do to Us

THE Florentines were probably mistaken in supposing
that their fellow citizen, Salvino degli Armati, was the
inventor of the lenses now so commonly worn to correct
errors of refraction. There has been much discussion
as to the origin of these devices, but they are generally
believed to have been known at a period much earlier
than that of Salvino degli Armati. The Romans at least
must have known something of the art of supplement-
ing the powers of the eye, for Pliny tells us that Nero
used to watch the games in the Colosseum through a
concave gem, set for that purpose in a ring. If, however,
his contemporaries believed that Salvino of the Armati
was the first to produce these aids to vision, they might
well have prayed for the pardon of his sins. While it is
true that eyeglasses have brought to some people
improved vision and relief from pain and discomfort,
they have been to others simply an added torture, they
always do more or less harm, and at their best they
never improve the vision to normal.

That glasses cannot improve the sight to normal can
be very simply demonstrated by looking at any colour
through a strong convex or concave glass. It will be
noted that the colour is always less intense than when
seen with the naked eye, and since the perception of

form depends upon the perception of colour, it follows that both colour and form must be less distinctly seen with glasses than without them. Even plane glass lowers the vision for both colour and form, as everyone knows who has ever looked out of a window. Women who wear glasses for minor defects of vision often observe that they are made more or less colour-blind by them, and in a shop one may note that they remove them when they want to match samples. However, if the sight is seriously defective, the colour may be seen better with glasses than without them.

That glasses must injure the eye is evident from the facts given in the preceding chapter. One cannot see through them unless one produces the degree of refractive error which they are designed to correct. But refractive errors, in the eye which is left to itself, are never constant. If one secures good vision by the aid of concave, convex, or astigmatic lenses, therefore, it means that one is maintaining constantly a degree of refractive error which otherwise would not be maintained constantly. It is only to be expected that this should make the condition worse, and it is a matter of common experience that it does.

After people once begin to wear glasses, their strength in most cases has to be steadily increased in order to maintain the degree of visual acuity secured by the aid of the first pair. Persons with presbyopia who put on glasses because they cannot read fine print too often find that after they have worn them for a time they cannot, without their aid, read the larger print that was perfectly plain to them before. A person with myopia of ·20/70 who puts on glasses giving him a vision of 20/20 may find that in a week's time his unaided vision has declined to 20/200. When people break their glasses and go without them for a week or two, they frequently observe that their sight has improved. As a matter of fact, the sight always improves to a greater or lesser degree when glasses are discarded, although the fact may not always be noted.

That the human eye resents glasses is a fact which no one would attempt to deny. Every oculist knows that patients have to 'get used' to them, and that sometimes they never succeed in doing so. Patients with high degrees of myopia and hypermetropia have great difficulty in accustoming themselves to the full correction, and often are never able to do so. The strong concave glasses required by myopes of high degree make all objects seem much smaller than they really are, while convex glasses enlarge them. These are unpleasantnesses that cannot be overcome. Patients with high degrees of astigmatism suffer some very disagreeable sensations when they first put on glasses, for which reason they are warned to get used to them at home before venturing out. Usually these difficulties are overcome, but often they are not, and it sometimes happens that those who get on fairly well with their glasses in the daytime never succeed in getting used to them at night.

All glasses contract the field of vision to a greater or lesser degree. Even with very weak glasses patients are unable to see distinctly unless they look through the centre of the lenses, with the frames at right angles to the line of vision; not only is their vision lowered if they fail to do this, but annoying nervous symptoms, such as dizziness and headache, are sometimes produced. Therefore they are unable to turn their eyes freely in different directions. It is true that glasses are now ground in such a way that it is theoretically possible to look through them at any angle, but practically they seldom accomplish the desired result.

The difficulty of keeping the glass clear is one of the minor discomforts of glasses, but it is nevertheless a most annoying one. On damp and rainy days the atmosphere clouds them. On hot days the perspiration from the body may have a similar effect. On cold days they are often clouded by the moisture of the breath. Every day they are so subject to contamination by dust and moisture and the touch of the fingers incident to unavoidable handling that they seldom afford an absolutely unobstructed view of the objects regarded.

Likewise, reflections of strong light from eyeglasses are often very annoying, and in the street may be very dangerous.

Soldiers, sailors, athletes, workmen and children have great difficulty with glasses because of the activity of their lives, which not only leads to the breaking of the lenses but often throws them out of focus, particularly in the case of eyeglasses worn for astigmatism.

The fact that glasses are very disfiguring may seem a matter unworthy of consideration here, but mental discomfort does not improve either the general health or the vision, and while we have gone so far toward making a virtue of what we conceive to be necessity that some persons have actually come to consider glasses becoming, there are still some unperverted minds to which the wearing of glasses is mental torture and the sight of them upon others far from agreeable. As for putting glasses upon a child, it is enough to make anyone sick at heart.

Upto a generation ago glasses were used only as an aid to defective sight, but they are now prescribed for large numbers of persons who can see as well or better without them. As explained in Chapter I, the hyper-metropic eye is believed to be capable of correcting its own difficulties to some extent by altering the curvature of the lens, through the activity of the ciliary muscle. The eye with simple myopia is not credited with this capacity, because an increase in the convexity of the lens, which is supposed to be all that is accomplished by accommodative effort, would only increase the difficulty; but myopia is usually accompanied by astigmatism, and this, it is believed, can be overcome in part by alterations in the curvature of the lens. Thus we are led by the theory to the conclusion that an eye in which any error of refraction exists is practically never free, while open, from abnormal accommodative efforts.

In other words, it is assumed that the supposed muscle of accommodation has to bear not only the normal burden of changing the focus of the eye for vision at different distances, but also the additional burden of compensating for refractive errors. Such adjustments, if they actually took place, would naturally impose a severe strain upon the nervous system, and it is to relieve this strain—which is believed to be the cause of a host of functional nervous troubles—quite as much as to improve the sight, that glasses are prescribed.

It has been demonstrated, however, that the lens is not a factor either in the production of accommodation or in the correction of errors of refraction. Therefore, under no circumstances can there be a strain of the ciliary muscle to be relieved. It has also been demonstrated that when the vision is normal no error of refraction is present, and the extrinsic (or external) muscles of the eyeball are at rest. Therefore there can be no strain of the extrinsic muscles to be relieved in these cases. When a strain of these muscles does exist, glasses may correct its effects upon the refraction, but the train itself they cannot relieve. On the contrary, as has been shown, they must make it worse.

Nevertheless, persons with normal vision who wear glasses for the relief of a supposed muscular strain are often benefitted by them. This is a striking illustration of the effect of mental suggestion, and plane glass, if it could inspire the same faith, would produce the same result. In fact, many patients have told me that they had been relieved of various discomforts by glasses which I found to be simply plane glass. One of these patients was an optician who had fitted the glasses himself and was under no illusions whatever about them, yet he assured me that when he didn't wear them he had headaches.

Some patients are so responsive to mental suggestion that you can relieve their discomfort or improve their sight with almost any glasses you like to put on them I have seen people with hypermetropia wearing myopic glasses with a great deal of comfort, and people with no astigmatism getting much satisfaction from glasses designed for the correction of this defect.

Many persons will even imagine that they see better with glasses that markedly lower the vision. A number of years ago a patient for whom I had prescribed glasses consulted an ophthalmologist whose reputation was much greater than my own and who gave him another pair of glasses and spoke slightingly of the ones that I had prescribed. The patient returned to me and told me how much better he could see with the second pair of glasses than he did with the first. I tested his vision with the new glasses, and found that while mine had given

39

him a vision of 20/20 those of my colleague enabled him to see only 20/40. The simple fact was that he had been hypnotized by a great reputation into thinking he could see better when he actually saw worse, and it was hard to convince him that he was wrong, although he had to admit that when he looked at the test card he could see only half as much with the new glasses as with the old ones.

When glasses do not relieve headaches and other nervous symptoms, it is assumed to be because they were not properly fitted, and some practitioners and their patients exhibit an astounding degree of patience and perseverance in their joint attempts to arrive at the proper prescription. A patient who suffered from severe pains at the base of his brain was fitted sixty times by one specialist alone, and had besides visited many other eye and nerve specialists in this country and in Europe. He was relieved of the pain in five minutes by the methods presented in this book, and at the same time his vision became temporarily normal.

It is fortunate that many people for whom glasses have been prescribed refuse to wear them, thus escaping not only much discomfort but also much injury to their eyes. Others, having less independence of mind or a larger share of the martyr's spirit, or having been more badly frightened by oculists, submit to an amount of unnecessary torture which is scarcely conceivable. One such patient wore glasses for twenty-five years, although they did not prevent her from suffering continual misery and lowered her vision to such an extent that she had to look over the tops when she wanted to see anything at a distance. Her oculist assured her that she might expect the most serious consequences if she did not wear the glasses, and was very severe about her

40

practice of looking over instead of through them.

As refractive abnormalities are continually changing from day to day, from hour to hour, and from minute to minute, even under the influence of atropine, the accurate fitting of glasses is, of course, impossible. In some cases these fluctuations are so extreme, or the patient is so unresponsive to mental suggestion, that no relief whatever is obtained from correcting lenses, which necessarily become an added discomfort. At their best it cannot be maintained that glasses are anything more than a very unsatisfactory substitute for normal vision.

6

The Cause and Treatment of Errors of Refraction

IT has been demonstrated in thousands of cases that all abnormal action of the external muscles of the eyeball is accompanied by a strain or effort to see, and that with the relief of this strain the action of the muscles become normal and all errors of refraction disappear. The eye may be blind, it may be suffering from atrophy of the optic nerve, from cataract, or from disease of the retina, but as long as it does not *try* to see, the external muscles act normally and there is no error of refraction. This fact furnishes us with the means by which all these conditions, so long held to be incurable, may be corrected.

It has also been demonstrated that for every error of refraction there is a different kind of strain. The study of images reflected from various parts of the eyeball confirmed what had previously been observed, namely, that myopia (or a lessening of hypermetropia) is always associated with a strain to see at the distance, while hypermetropia (or a lessening of myopia) is always associated with a strain to see at the near-point. These facts can be verified in a few minutes by anyone who knows how to use a retinoscope, provided only that the instrument is not brought nearer to the subject than six feet.

In an eye with previously normal vision a strain to see near objects always results in the temporary production of hypermetropia in one or all meridians. That is, the eye either becomes entirely hypermetropic or some form of astigmatism is produced of which hypermetropia forms a part. In the hypermetropic eye the hypermetropia is increased in one or all meridians. When the myopic eye strains to see a near object the myopia is lessened and emmetropia (that condition of the eye in which it is focused for parallel rays, which constitutes normal vision at the distance but is an error of refraction when it occurs at the near-point) may be produced, the eye being focused for the far-point while still trying to see at the near-point. In some cases the emmetropia may even pass over into hypermetropia in one or all meridians. All these changes are accompanied by evidences of increasing strain and lowered vision (see Chapter 8), but strange to say, pain and fatigue are usually relieved to a marked degree.

If, on the other hand, the eye with previously normal vision strains to see at the distance, temporary myopia is always produced in one or all meridians, and if the eye is already myopic, the myopia is increased. If the hypermetropic eye strains to see a distant object, pain and fatigue may be produced or increased, but the hypermetropia is lessened and the vision improved. This interesting result, it will be noted, is the exact opposite of what we get when the myope strains to see at the near-point. In some cases the hypermetropia is completely relieved and emmetropia is produced, with a complete disappearance of all evidences of strain. This condition may then pass over into myopia, with an increase of strain as the myopia increases.

In other words, the eye which strains to see at the near-point becomes flatter than it was before, in one or all meridians. If it was elongated to start with, it may pass from this condition through emmetropia, in which it is spherical, to hypermetropia, in which it is flattened and if these changes take place unsymmetrically, astigmatism will be produced in connection with the other conditions. The eye which strains to see at the distance, on the contrary, becomes rounder than it was before and may pass from the flattened condition of hypermetropia, through emmetropia, to the elongated condition of myopia. If these changes take place unsymmetrically, astigmatism will again be produced in connection with the other conditions.

What has been said of the normal eye applies equally to eyes from which the lens has been removed. This operation usually produces a condition of hypermetropia, but when there has previously been a condition of high myopia the removal of the lens may not be sufficient to correct it and the eye may still remain myopic. In the first case a strain to see at the distance lessens the hypermetropia and a strain to see at the near-point increases it; in the second a strain to see at the distance increases the myopia and a strain to see at the near-point lessens it. Many aphakic, or lensless, eyes strain to see at the near-point for a longer or shorter period after the removal of the lens, producing so much hypermetropia that the patient cannot read ordinary print, and the power of accommodation appears to be completely lost. Later, when the patient becomes accustomed to the situation, this strain is often relieved and the eye becomes able to focus accurately upon near objects. Some rare cases have also been observed in which a measure of good vision both for distance and the near-point was obtained without glasses, the eyeball elongating sufficiently to, compensate, to some degree, for the loss of the lens.

The phenomena associated with strain in the human eye have also been observed in the eye of the lower animals. I have made many dogs myopic by inducing them to strain to see a distant object. One very nervous dog, with normal refraction as demonstrated by the retinoscope, was allowed to smell a piece of meat. He became very much excited, pricked up his ears, arched his eyebrows and wagged his tail. The meat was then removed to a distance of twenty feet. The dog looked disappointed, but did not lose interest. While he was watching the meat it was dropped into a box. A worried look came into his eyes. He strained to see what had become of the meat, and the retinoscope showed that he had become myopic. This experiment, it should be added, would succeed only with an animal possessing two active oblique muscles. Animals in which one of these muscles is absent or rudimentary are unable to elongate the eyeball under any circumstances.

Primarily, the strain to see is a strain of the mind, and as in all cases in which there is a strain of the mind, there is a loss of mental control. Anatomically, the results of straining to see at a distance may be the same as those of regarding an object at the near-point without strain, but in one case the eye does what the mind desires and in the other it does not.

These facts appear to explain sufficiently why vision declines as civilization advances. Under the conditions of civilized life men's minds are under a continual strain. They have more things to worry them than

45

uncivilized man had, and they are not obliged to keep cool and collected in order that they may see and do other things upon which existence depends. If he allowed himself to get nervous, primitive man was promptly eliminated, but civilized man survives and transmits his mental characteristics to posterity. The lower animals when subjected to civilized conditions respond to them in precisely the same way as human creatures. I have examined many domestic and menagerie animals, and have found them in many cases myopic, although they neither read, write, sew, nor set type.

A decline in vision at the distance, however, is no more a peculiarity of civilization than is a similar decline at the near-point. Myopes, although they see better at the near-point than they do at the distance, never see as well as does the eye with normal sight; and in hypermetropia, which is more common than myopia, the sight is worse at the near-point than at the distance.

The remedy is not to avoid either near work or distant vision, but to get rid of the mental strain which underlies the imperfect functioning of the eye at both points. It has been demonstrated in thousands of cases that this can be done.

Fortunately, all persons are able to relax under certain conditions at will. In all uncomplicated errors of refraction the strain to see can be relieved, temporarily, by having the patient look at a blank wall without trying to see. To secure permanent relaxation sometimes requires considerable time and much ingenuity. The same method cannot be used with everyone. The ways in which people strain to see are infinite, and the methods used to relieve the strain must be almost equally

46

varied. Whatever the method that brings most relief, however, the end is always the same, namely, relaxation. By constant repetition and frequent demonstration and by all means possible, the fact must be stressed that perfect sight can be obtained only by relaxation.

Most people, when told that rest or relaxation will cure their eye troubles, ask why sleep does not do so. The answer to this question was given in Chapter 4. The eyes are rarely, if ever, completely relaxed in sleep, and if they are under a strain when the subject is awake, the strain will certainly be continued during sleep to a greater or lesser degree, just as a strain of other parts of the body is continued.

The idea that it rests the eyes not to use them is also erroneous. The eyes were made to see with, and if when they are open they do not see, it is because they are under such a strain and have such a great error of refraction that they cannot see. Near vision, although accomplished by a muscular act, is no more a strain on them than is distant vision, which is accomplished without the intervention of the muscles. The use of the muscles does not necessarily produce fatigue. Some men can run for hours without becoming tired. Many birds support themselves upon one foot during sleep, the toes tightly clasping the swaying bough and the muscles remaining unfatigued by the apparent strain.

The fact is that when the mind is at rest nothing can tire the eyes, and when the mind is under a strain nothing can rest them. Anything that rests the mind will benefit the eyes. Almost everyone has observed that the eyes tire less quickly when reading an interesting book than when reading something tiresome or difficult to comprehend. A schoolboy can sit up all night reading a novel without even thinking of his eyes, but if he tried to sit up all night studying his lessons he would soon find his eyes getting very tired. A child whose vision was ordinarily so acute that she could see the moons of Jupiter with the naked eye became myopic when asked to do a sum in mental arithmetic, mathematics being a subject which was extremely distasteful to her.

Sometimes the conditions which produce mental relaxation are very curious. One woman, for instance, was able to correct her error of refraction when she looked at the test card with her body bent over at an angle of about forty-five degrees, and the relaxation continued after she had assumed an upright position. Although the position was an unfavourable one, she had somehow got the idea that it improved her sight, and therefore it did so.

The time required to effect a permanent improvement varies greatly with different individuals. In some cases five, or fifteen minutes is sufficient, and I believe the time is coming when it will be possible to relieve everyone quickly. It is only a question of accumulating more facts and presenting these facts in such a way that they may be grasped quickly. At present, however, it is often necessary to continue treatment for weeks and months, although the error of refraction may be no greater and of no longer duration than in those cases that are cured quickly.

In most cases, too the treatment must be continued for a few minutes every day to prevent relapse. Because a familiar object tends to relax the strain to see, the daily reading of a test card is usually sufficient for this purpose. It is also useful, particularly when vision at the near-point is imperfect, to read fine print every day as close to the eyes as it can be done. When the improvement is complete it is always permanent—nevertheless, the attainment not of what is ordinarily called normal sight but of a measure to telescopic and microscopic vision is very rare. Even in these cases, too, the treatment can be continued with benefit: it is impossible to place limits on the visual powers of man; and no matter how good the sight, it is always possible to improve it.

Daily practice of the art of vision is also necessary to prevent those visual lapses to which every eye is liable, no matter how good its sight may be ordinarily. It is true that no system of training will provide an absolute safeguard against such lapses in all circumstances, but the daily reading of small, distant, familiar letters will do much to lessen the tendency to strain when disturbing circumstances arise, and all persons upon whose eyesight the safety of others depends should be required to do this.

Generally, persons who have never worn glasses are more easily relieved than those who have, and glasses should be discarded as the beginning of the treatment. When this cannot be done without too great discomfort, or when a person has to continue his work during the treatment and cannot do so without glasses, their use must be permitted for a time—but this always delays improvement. Persons of all ages have been benefitted by this treatment of errors of refraction by relaxation, but children usually, though not invariably, respond much more quickly than adults. If they are under twelve years of age, or even under sixteen, and have never worn glasses, the condition is usually eliminated in a few days, weeks, or months, and always within a year, simply by reading a test card every day.

7

Strain

TEMPORARY conditions may contribute to the strain to
see which results in the production of errors of refraction, but its foundation lies in wrong habits of thought.
In attempting to relieve it, the physician has to struggle
continually against the idea that to do anything well
requires effort. This idea is drilled into us from our
cradles. The whole educational system is based upon it,
and educators who call themselves modern still cling to
the club, under various disguises, as a necessary
auxiliary to the process of teaching.

It is as natural for the eye to see as it is for the mind
to acquire knowledge, and any effort in either case not
only is useless but defeats the end in view. You may
force a few facts into a child's mind by various kinds
of compulsion, but you cannot make him learn anything.
The facts remain, if they remain at all, as dead lumber
in the brain. They contribute nothing to the vital
processes of thought, and because they are not acquired
naturally and are not assimilated, they destroy the
natural impulse of the mind toward the acquisition of
knowledge. By the time the child leaves school or
college, as the case may be, he not only knows nothing
but is, in the majority of cases, no longer capable of
learning.

In the same way you may temporarily improve the sight by effort, but you cannot improve it to normal, and if the effort is allowed to become continuous, the sight will steadily deteriorate and may eventually be destroyed. Very seldom is the impairment or destruction of vision due to any fault in the construction of the eye. Of two equally good pairs of eyes, one will retain perfect sight to the end of life and the other will lose it in the kindergarten, simply because one looks at things without effort and the other does not.

The eye with normal sight never *tries* to see. If for any reason—the dimness of the light, for instance, or the distance of the object—it cannot see a particular point, it shifts to another. It never tries to bring out the point by staring at it, as the eye with imperfect sight is constantly doing.

Whenever the eye tries to see, it at once ceases to have normal vision. A person may look at the stars with normal vision, but if he tries to count the stars in any particular constellation he will probably become myopic, because the attempt usually results in an effort to see. A patient was able to look at the letter K on a test card with normal vision, but when asked to count the twenty-seven corners which that letter happened to have, he lost it completely.

It obviously requires a strain to fail to see at the distance, because, as I have already stated, the eye at rest is adjusted for distant vision. If one does anything when one wants to see at the distance, it must be the wrong thing. The shape of the eyeball cannot be altered during distant vision without strain. It is equally a strain to fail to see at the near-point, because when the muscles respond to the mind's desire they do it without strain. Only by an effort can one prevent the eye from elongating at the near-point.

The eye possesses 'perfect vision' only when it is absolutely at rest. Any movement, either in the organ or the object of vision, produces an error of refraction. With the retinoscope it can be demonstrated that even the necessary movements of the eyeball produce a slight error of refraction, and the motion picture has given us a practical demonstration of the fact that it is impossible to see a moving object perfectly. When the movement of the object seen is sufficiently slow, the resulting impairment of vision is so slight as to be inappreciable, just as the errors of refraction produced by slight movements of the eyeball are inappreciable, but when objects move very rapidly they can be seen only as a blur. For this reason it has been found necessary to arrange the machinery for exhibiting motion pictures in such a way that each picture is halted for one sixteenth of a second and screened while it is moving into place. Motion pictures, accordingly, are never seen actually in motion.

The act of seeing is passive. Things are seen, just as they are felt or heard or tasted, without effort or volition on the part of the subject. When sight is perfect the letters on the test card are waiting, perfectly black and perfectly distinct, to be recognized. They do not have to be sought; they are there. In imperfect sight they are sought and chased. The eye goes after them. An effort is made to see them.

The muscles of the body are supposed never to be at rest. The blood vessels, with their muscular coats, are never at rest. Even in sleep thought does not cease. But the normal condition of the nerves of sense—of hearing, sight, taste, smell and touch is one of rest. They can be acted upon; they cannot act. The optic nerve, the retina and the visual centres of the brain are as passive as the fingernail. They have nothing whatever in their structure that makes it possible for them to do anything, and when they are the subject of effort from outside sources their efficiency is always impaired.

The mind is the source of all such efforts from outside sources brought to bear upon the eye. Every thought of effort in the mind, of whatever sort, transmits a motor impulse to the eye, and every such impulse causes a deviation from the normal in the shape of the eyeball and lessens the sensitiveness of the centre of sight. If one wants to avoid errors of refraction, therefore, one must have no thought of effort in the mind. Mental strain of any kind always produces a conscious or unconscious eyestrain, and if the strain takes the form of an effort to see, an error of refraction is always produced.

A schoolboy who came to my notice was able to read the bottom line of the Snellen test card at ten feet, but when the teacher told him to mind what he was about he could not see the big C, which is normally read at two hundred feet. Many children can see perfectly as long as their mothers are around, but if the mother goes out of the room they may at once become myopic, because of the strain produced by fear. Unfamiliar objects produce eye-strain and a consequent error of refraction because they first produce mental strain. A person may have good vision when he is telling the truth; but if he states what is not true, even with no intent to deceive, or if he imagines what is not true, an error of refraction will be produced, because it is impossible to state or imagine what is not true without an effort.

I may claim to have discovered that telling lies is bad for the eyes, and whatever bearing this circumstance may have upon the universality of defects of vision, the fact can easily be demonstrated. If a person can read all the small letters on the bottom line of the test card and either deliberately or carelessly miscalls any of them, the retinoscope will indicate an error of refraction. In numerous cases people have been asked to state their ages incorrectly, or to try to imagine that they were a year older or a year younger than they actually were, and always the retinoscope indicated an error of refraction. A man twenty-five years old had no error of refraction when he looked at a blank wall without trying to see, but if he said he was twenty-six or if someone else said he was twenty-six, or if he tried to imagine that he was twenty-six, he became myopic. The same thing happened when he stated or tried to imagine that he was twenty-four. When he stated or remembered the truth his vision was normal, but when he stated or imagined an error he had an error of refraction.

Mental strain may produce many different kinds of eyestrain. According to the statement of most authorities there is only one kind of eyestrain, an indefinite thing resulting from so-called over-use of the eyes, or an effort to overcome a wrong shape of the eyeball. It can be demonstrated, however, that there is not only a different strain for each different error of refraction but a different strain for most abnormal conditions of the eye. The strain that produces an error of refraction is not the same as the strain that produces a squint, a cataract, glaucoma (a condition in which the eyeball becomes abnormally hard), amblyopia, inflammation of the conjuctiva (a membrane covering the inner surface of the eyelid and the visible part of the white of the eye) or of the margin of the lids, or disease of the optic nerve or retina.

All these conditions may exist with only a slight error of refraction, and while the relief of one strain usually means the relief of any others that may coexist with it, it sometimes happens that the strain associated with such conditions as cataract and glaucoma is relieved without the complete relief of the strain that causes the error of refraction. Even the pain that so often accompanies errors of refraction is never caused by the same strain that causes these errors. Some myopes cannot read without pain or discomfort, but most of them suffer no inconvenience. When the hypermetrope regards an object at the distance, the hypermetropia is lessened but pain and discomfort may be increased. While there are many strains, however, there is only one cure for all of them—relaxation.

The health of the eye depends upon the blood, and circulation is very largely influenced by thought. When thought is normal—that is, not attended by any excitement or strain—the circulation in the brain is normal, the supply of blood to the optic nerve and the visual centres is normal, and the vision is normal. When thought is abnormal the circulation is disturbed, the supply of blood to the optic nerve and visual centres is altered and the vision is lowered. We can consciously think thoughts which disturb the circulation and lower the visual power; we can also consciously think thoughts that will restore normal circulation and thereby help to cure errors of refraction and many other abnormal conditions of the eyes. We cannot by any amount of effort make ourselves see, but by learning to control our thoughts we can accomplish the end indirectly.

You can teach people how to produce any error of refraction, how to produce a squint, how to see two images of an object, one above another or side by side or at any desired angle from one another, simply by teaching them how to think in a particular way. When the disturbing thought is replaced by one that relaxes, the squint disappears and the double vision and the errors of refraction are corrected; this is as true of abnormalities of long standing as it is of those produced voluntarily. No matter what their degree or their duration, their elimination is accomplished just as soon as the patient is able to secure mental control. The origin of any error of refraction, of a squint, or of any other functional disturbance of the eye, is simply a thought—a wrong thought—and its disappearance is as quick as the thought that relaxes. In a fraction of a second the highest degree of refractive error may be corrected, a squint may disappear, or the blindness of amblyopia may be relieved. If the relaxation is only momentary, the correction is momentary. When it becomes permanent, the correction is permanent.

This relaxation cannot, however, be obtained by any sort of *effort*. It is fundamental that a person should understand this; so long as he thinks, consciously or unconsciously, that relief from strain may be obtained by another strain, the improvement will be delayed.

8

Central Fixation

THE eye is a miniature camera, corresponding in many ways very exactly to the inanimate machine used in photography. In one respect, however, there is a great difference between the two instruments. The sensitive plate of the camera is equally sensitive in every part; the retina of the eye, on the other hand, has a point of maximum sensitiveness, and every other part is less sensitive in proportion to its distance from that point. This point of maximum sensitiveness is called the *fovea centralis*, literally the 'central pit'.

The retina, although it is an extremely delicate membrane varying in thickness from one-eightieth of an inch to less than half that amount, is highly complex. It is composed of eight layers, only one of which is supposed to be capable of receiving visual impressions. This layer is composed of minute rodlike and conical bodies which vary in form and are distributed very differently in its different parts. In the centre of the retina is a small circular elevation known, from the yellow colour which it assumes in death and sometimes also in life, as the *macula lutea*, literally the 'yellow spot'. In the centre of this spot is the fovea, a deep depression of darker colour. In the centre of this depression there are no rods and the cones are elongated

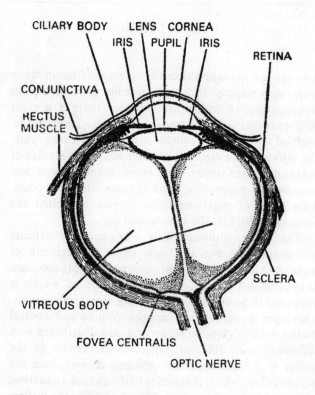

CILIARY BODY   LENS CORNEA

IRIS   PUPIL IRIS

RETINA

CONJUNCTIVA

RECTUS
MUSCLE

SCLERA

VITREOUS BODY

FOVEA CENTRALIS

OPTIC NERVE

Horizontal Section of the Eyeball

and pressed very closely together. The other layers, on the contrary, become extremely thin here or disappear altogether, so that the cones are covered with barely perceptible traces of them. Beyond the centre of the fovea the cones become thicker and fewer and are interspersed with rods, the number of which increases toward the margin of the retina.

The precise function of these rods and cones is not clear, but it is a fact that the centre of the fovea, where all elements except the cones and their associated cells practically disappear, is the seat of the most acute vision. As we withdraw from this spot the acuteness of the visual perceptions rapidly decreases. The eye with normal vision, therefore, sees one part of everything it looks at best, and all other parts worse, in proportion to their distance from the point of maximum vision; and it is an invariable symptom of all abnormal conditions of the eyes, both functional and organic, that this *central fixation* is lost.

These conditions are due to the fact that when the sight is normal, the sensitiveness of the fovea is normal, but when the sight is imperfect, from whatever cause, the sensitiveness of the fovea is lowered so that the eye sees just as well, or even better, with other parts of the retina. Contrary to what is generally believed, the part seen best when the sight is normal is extremely small. The textbooks say that at twenty feet an area having a diameter of half an inch can be seen with maximum vision, but anyone who tries at this distance to see every part of even the smallest letters of the Snellen test card—and their diameter may be less than a quarter of an inch—equally well at one time will immediately become myopic. The fact is that the nearer the point of maximum vision approaches a mathematical point, which has no area, the better the sight.

The cause of this loss of function in the centre of sight is mental strain; and as all abnormal conditions of the eyes, organic as well as functional, are accompanied by mental strain, all conditions must necessarily be accompanied by loss of central fixation. When the mind is under a strain the eye usually goes more or less blind. The centre of sight goes blind first, partially or completely, according to the degree of the strain, and if the strain is great enough the whole or the greater part of the retina may be involved. When the vision of the centre of sight has been suppressed, partially or completely, a person can no longer see best the point at which he is looking——he sees objects not regarded directly as well, or better, because the sensitiveness of the retina has now become approximately equal in every part or is even better in the outer part than in the centre. Therefore in all cases of defective vision a person is unable to see best where he is looking.

This condition is sometimes so extreme that a person may look as far away from an object as it is possible to see it, and yet see it just as well as when he is looking directly at it. In one case this had gone so far that a patient of mine could see only with the edge of the retina on the nasal side. In other words, she could not see her fingers in front of her face, but could see them if they were held at the outer side of her eye. She had only a slight error of refraction, showing that while every error of refraction is accompanied by eccentric fixation, the strain which causes the one condition is different from that which produces the other. The patient had been examined by specialists in this country and Europe, who attributed her blindness to disease of the optic nerve or brain; the fact that vision was restored by relaxation demonstrated that the condition had been due simply to mental strain.

Economic fixation, even in its lesser degrees, is so un-natural that great discomfort and pain can be produced in a few seconds by trying to see every part of an area three or four inches in extent at twenty feet, or even less, or an area of an inch or less at the near-point, equally well at one time. At the same time the retinoscope will demonstrate that an error of refraction has been produced. This strain, when it is habitual, leads to all sorts of abnormal conditions and is, in fact, at the bottom of most eye troubles, both functional and organic. The discomfort and pain may be absent however, in the chronic condition, and thus it is an encouraging sign when a person begins to experience them.

When the eye possesses central fixation, it not only possesses impeccable sight but is perfectly at rest and can be used indefinitely without fatigue. It is open and quiet, no nervous movements are observable, and when it regards a point at a distance the visual axes are parallel. In other words, there are no muscular insufficiencies. This fact is not generally known. The textbooks state that muscular insufficiencies occur in eyes having normal sight, but I have never seen such a case. The muscles of the face and of the whole body are also at rest, and when the condition is habitual there are no wrinkles or dark circles around the eyes.

In most cases of economic fixation, on the contrary, the eye quickly tires and its appearance, with that of the face, is expressive of effort or strain. The ophthalmoscope (an instrument with which we can see the interior of the eye) reveals that the eyeball moves

61

at irregular intervals, from side to side, vertically or in other directions.* These movements are often so extensive as to be revealed by ordinary inspection, and are sometimes sufficiently marked to resemble nystagmus (a condition in which there is a conspicuous and more or less rhythmic movement of the eyeball from side to side). Nervous movements of the eyelids may also be noted, either by ordinary inspection or by lightly touching the lid of one eye while the other regards an object either at the near-point or the distance. The visual axes are never parallel, and the deviation from the normal may become so marked as to constitute the condition of squint. Redness of the conjuctiva and of the margins of the lids, wrinkles around the eyes, dark circles beneath them, and tearing are other symptoms of eccentric fixation.

Eccentric fixation is a symptom of strain and is relieved by any method that relieves strain, but in some cases a person is relieved just as soon as he is able to demonstrate the facts of central fixation. When he comes to realize, through actual demonstration of the fact, that he does not see best where he is looking, but that when he looks a sufficient distance away from a point he can see it *worse* than when he looks directly at it, he becomes able, in some way, to reduce the distance to which he has to look in order to see worse, until he can look directly at the top of a small letter and see the bottom worse, or look at the bottom and see the top worse.

*A shorter movement can be noted when the observer watches the optic nerve with the ophthalmoscope than when he views merely the exterior of the eye.

The smaller the letter regarded in this way, or the shorter the distance the patient has to look away from a letter in order to see the opposite part indistinctly, the greater the relaxation and the better the sight. When it becomes possible to look at the bottom of a letter and see the top worse, or to look at the top and see the bottom worse, it becomes possible to see the letter perfectly black and distinct. At first such vision may come only in flashes: the letter will come out distinctly for a moment and then disappear. But gradually, if the practice is continued, central fixation will become habitual.

Most people can readily look at the bottom of the big C on a test and see the top of the letter worse, but in some cases it is not only impossible for them to do this but impossible for them to let go of the large letters at any distance at which they can be seen. These extreme cases sometimes require considerable ingenuity, first to demonstrate to a person that he does not see best where he is looking, and then to help him to see an object worse when he looks away from it than when he looks directly at it. The use of a strong light as one of the points of fixation, or of two lights five or ten feet apart, has been found helpful. A person when he looks away from the light will be able to see it less bright more readily than he can see a black letter worse when he looks away from it. It then becomes easier for him to see the letter worse when he looks away from it. This method was successful in the following case.

A woman with vision of 3/200 said she saw the big C better when she looked at a point a few feet away from it than when she looked directly at it. Her attention was called to the fact that her eyes soon became tired and that her vision soon failed when she saw things this way. Then she was directed to look at a bright object about three feet away from the card, and this attracted her attention to such an extent that she became able to see the large letter on the test card worse, after which she was able to look back at it and see it better. It was demonstrated to her that she could do one of two things: look away and see the letter better than she did before, or look away and see it worse. She then became able to see it worse all the time when she looked three feet away from it. Next she became able to shorten the distance successively to two feet, one foot, and six inches, with a constant improvement in vision. Finally she could look at the bottom of the letter and see the top worse, or look at the top and see the bottom worse. With practice she became able to look at the smaller letters in the same way, and finally she read the ten line (the line that should normally be read at ten feet) at twenty feet. By the same method also she was enabled to read diamond type first at twelve inches and then at three inches. By these simple measures alone she became able, in short, to see best where she was looking, and her recovery was complete.

The highest degrees of eccentric fixation occur in the high degrees of myopia, and in these cases, since the sight is best at the near-point, a person is benefitted by practising seeing worse at this point. The distance can then be gradually extended until it becomes possible to do the same thing at twenty feet. One of my patients with a high degree of myopia said that the father she looked away from an electric light the better she saw it, but by alternately looking at the light at the near-point and looking away from it she became able, in a short time, to see it brighter when she looked directly at it than when she looked away from it. Later she became able to do the same thing at twenty feet, and then she experienced a great feeling of relief. No words, she said, could adequately describe it. Every nerve seemed to be relaxed, and a feeling of comfort and rest permeated her whole body. Afterward her progress was rapid. She soon became able to look at one part of the smallest letters on the card and see the rest worse, and then she became able to read the letters at twenty feet.

On the principle that a burnt child dreads the fire, some people are benefitted by consciously making their sight worse. When they learn, by actual demonstration of the facts, just how their visual defects are produced, they unconsciously avoid the unconscious strain which causes them. When the degree of eccentric fixation is not too extreme to be increased, therefore, it is of benefit to learn how to increase it. When a person has consciously lowered his vision and produced discomfort and even pain by trying to see the big C, or a whole line of letters, equally well at one time, he becomes better able to correct the unconscious effort of the eye to see all parts of a small area equally well at one time.

In learning to see best where he is looking, it is usually best for a person to think of the point not directly regarded as being seen less distinctly than the point he is looking at, instead of thinking of the point fixed as being seen best, as the latter practice has a tendency in most cases to intensify the strain under which the eye is already laboring. One part of an object is seen best only when the mind is content to see the greater part of it indistinctly, and as the degree of relaxation increases, the area of the part seen worse increases, until that seen best becomes merely a point.

The limits of vision depend upon the degree of central fixation. A person may be able to read a sign half a mile away when he sees the letters all alike, but when taught to see one letter best he will be able to read smaller letters that he didn't know were there. The remarkable vision of savages, who can see with the naked eye objects for which most civilized persons require a telescope, is a matter of central fixation. Some people can see the rings of Saturn or the moons of Jupiter with the naked eye. It is not because of any superiority in the structure of their eyes, but because they have attained a higher degree of central fixation than most civilized persons do.

Not only do all errors of refraction and all functional disturbances of the eye disappear when it sees by central fixation, but many organic conditions are relieved. I am unable to set any limits to its possibilities. I would not have ventured to predict that glaucoma, incipient cataract, and syphilitic iritis (inflammation of the iris of the eye) could be eliminated by central fixation, but it is a fact that these conditions have disappeared when central fixation was attained. Relief was often obtained in a few minutes, and, in rare cases, this relief was permanent. Usually, however, a permanent improvement required more prolonged treatment. Inflammatory conditions of all kinds, including inflammation of the cornea, iris, conjuctiva, the various coats of the eyeball and even the optic nerve itself, have been benefitted by central fixation after other methods have failed. Infections, as well as diseases caused by protein poisoning and the poisons of typhoid fever, influenza, syphilis and gonorrhoea,

66

have also been benefitted by it. Even with a foreign body in the eye there is no redness and no pain so long as central fixation is retained.

Since central fixation is impossible without mental control, central fixation of the eye means central fixation of the mind. It means, therefore, health in all parts of the body, for all the operations of the physical mechanism depend upon the mind. Not merely the sight, but all the other senses—touch, taste, hearing, and smell—are benefitted by central fixation. All the vital processes—digestion, assimilation, elimination, etc—are improved by it. The symptoms of functional and organic diseases are relieved. The efficiency of the mind is enormously increased. The benefits of central fixation already observed are, in short, so great that the subject merits further investigation.

⑨

Palming

ALL the methods used in the eradication of errors of refraction are simply different ways of obtaining relaxation, and most people, though by no means all, find it easiest to relax with their eyes shut. This usually lessens the strain to see, and in such cases is followed by a temporary or more lasting improvement in vision.

Most people are benefitted merely by closing the eyes; and by alternately resting them for a few minutes or longer in this way and then opening them and looking at a test card for a second or less, flashes of improved vision are as a rule very quickly obtained. Some temporarily obtain almost normal vision by this means, and in rare cases a complete restoration has been effected, sometimes in less than an hour.

But some light comes through the closed eyelids, and a still greater degree of relaxation can be obtained, in all but a few exceptional cases, by excluding it. This is done by covering the closed eyes with the palms of the hand (the fingers being crossed upon the forehead) in such a way as to avoid pressure on the eyeballs. So efficacious is this practice, which I have called 'palming', as a means of relieving strain, that we all instinctively respond to it at times, and from it most people are able to get a considerable degree of relaxation.

But even with the eyes closed and covered in such a way as to exclude all the light, the visual centres of the brain may still be disturbed, the eye may still strain to see; and instead of seeing a field so black that it is impossible to remember, imagine, or see anything blacker, as one ought normally to do when the optic nerve is not subject to the stimulation of light, a person will see illusions of lights and colour ranging all the way from an imperfect black to kaleidoscopic appearances so vivid that they seem to be actually seen with the eyes. The worse the condition of the eyesight, as a rule, the more numerous, vivid, and persistent these appearances are. Yet some persons with very imperfect sight are able to palm almost perfectly from the beginning, and are therefore very quickly relieved. Any disturbance of mind or body, such as fatigue, hunger, anger, worry or depression, also makes it difficult for patients to see black when they palm, persons who can see it perfectly under ordinary conditions often being unable to do so without assistance when they are ill or in pain.

It is impossible to see a perfect black unless the eyesight is faultless, because only then is the mind at rest; but some people can without difficulty approximate such a black nearly enough to improve their eyesight, and as the eyesight improves the deepness of the black increases. People who fail to see even an approximate black when they palm state that instead of black they see streaks or floating clouds of grey, flashes of light, patches of red, blue, green, yellow, etc. Sometimes instead of an immovable black, clouds of black will be seen moving across the field. In other cases the black will be seen for a few seconds and then some other colour will take its place. The different ways in which people can fail to see black when their eyes are closed and

69

covered are, in fact, very numerous and often very peculiar.

Some people have been so impressed with the vividness of the colours which they imagined they saw that no amount of argument could, or did, convince them that they did not actually see them with their eyes. If other people saw bright lights or colours with their eyes closed and covered, they admitted that these things would be illusions, but what they themselves saw under the same conditions was reality. They would not believe, until they had themselves demonstrated the truth, that their illusions were due to an imagination beyond their control.

Successful palming in these more difficult cases usually involves the practice of all the methods for improving the sight described in succeeding chapters. For reasons which will be explained in the following chapter, the majority of such people may be greatly helped by the memory of a black object. They should look at such an object at the distance at which the colour can be seen best, close the eyes and remember the colour, and repeat until the memory appears to be equal to the sight. Then, while still holding the memory of the black, they should cover the closed eyes with the palms of the hands in the manner just described. If the memory of the black is perfect, the whole background will be black. If it is not, or if it does not become so in the course of a few seconds, the eyes should be opened and the black object regarded again.

Many persons become able by this method to see black almost perfectly for a short time, but most of them, even those whose eyes are not very bad, have great difficulty in seeing it continuously. Being unable to remember black for more than three to five seconds

70

they cannot see black for a longer time than this. Such persons are helped by central fixation. When they have become able to see one part of a black object darker than the whole, they are able to remember the smaller area for a longer time than they could the larger one, and thus become able to see black for a longer period when they palm. They are also benefitted by mentally shifting (see Chapter 12) from one black object to another, or from one part of a black object to another.

It is impossible to see, remember, or imagine anything, even for as much as a second, without shifting from one part to another, or to some other object and back again, and the attempt to do so always produces strain. Those who think they are remembering a black object continuously are unconsciously comparing it with something not so black, or else its colour and its position are constantly changing. It is impossible to remember even such a simple thing as a full stop perfectly black and stationary for more than a fraction of a second.

When shifting is not done unconsciously it must be done consciously. For instance, remember successively a black hat, a black shoe, a black velvet dress, a black plush curtain, or a fold in the black dress or the black curtain, holding each one not more than a fraction of a second. Many persons have been benefitted by remembering all the letters of the alphabet in turn perfectly black. Others prefer to shift from one small black object, such as a full stop or a small letter, to another, or to 'swing' such an object in a manner to be described later (see Chapter 12).

In some cases the following method has proved successful. When a person sees what he thinks is a perfect black, let him remember a piece of white chalk on this background, and on the chalk the letter F as black as the background. Then let him forget the chalk and remember only the F, one part best, on the black background. In a short time the whole field may become as black as the blacker part of the F. The process can be repeated many times with a constant increase of blackness in the field.

In one case a woman who saw grey so vividly when she palmed that she was positive that she saw it with her eyes, instead of merely imagining it, was able to obliterate nearly all of it by first imagining a black C on the grey field, then two black C's, and finally a multitude of overlapping C's.

It is impossible to remember black perfectly when it is not seen perfectly. If one sees it imperfectly, the best one can do is to remember it imperfectly. All persons, without exception, who can see or read diamond type at the nearpoint, no matter how great their myopia may be or how much the interior of the eye may be diseased, can become able to see black with their eyes closed and covered more readily than persons with hypermetropia or astigmatism. This is because myopes, while they cannot see anything perfectly even at the near-point, see better at that point than persons with hypermetropia or astigmatism do at any distance. Persons with high degrees of myopia, however, often find palming very difficult, since they not only see black very imperfectly but, because of the effort they are making to see, cannot remember it for more than one or two seconds.

Any other condition of the eye which prevents a person from seeing black perfectly also makes palming difficult. In some cases black is never seen as black, appearing to be grey, yellow, brown, or even bright red. In such cases it is usually best to improve the sight by other methods to be described later, before trying to palm. Blind persons usually have more trouble in seeing black than those who can see, but they may be helped by the memory of a black object familiar to them before they lost their sight. A blind painter who saw grey continually when he first tried to palm became able at last to see black by the aid of the memory of black paint. He had no perception whatever of light and was in terrible pain, but when he succeeded in seeing black the pain vanished, and when he opened his eyes he saw light.

Even the imperfect memory of black is useful, for by its aid a still blacker black can be both remembered and seen, and this brings still further improvement. For instance, regard a letter on a test card at the distance at which the colour is seen best, then close the eyes and remember it. If the palming produces relaxation, it will be possible to imagine a deeper shade of black than was seen, and by remembering this black when again regarding the letter it can be seen blacker than it was at first. A still deeper black can then be imagined, and this deeper black can in turn be transferred to the letter on the test card. By continuing this process a perfect perception of black, and hence perfect sight, is sometimes very quickly obtained. The deeper the shade of black imagined with the eyes closed, the more easily it can be remembered when regarding the letters on the test card.

The longer some people palm the greater the relaxation they obtain and the darker the shade of black they are able both to remember and see. Others, it should be noted, are able to palm successfully for short periods but begin to strain if they keep it up too long.

It is impossible to succeed by effort, or by attempting to 'concentrate' on the black. As popularly understood, concentration means to do or think one thing only—but this is impossible and an attempt to do the impossible is a strain which defeats its own end. The human mind is not capable of thinking of one thing only. It can think of one thing best, and is at rest only when it does so, but it cannot think of one thing only. A woman who tried to see black only and to ignore the kaleidoscopic colours which intruded themselves upon her field of vision, becoming worse and worse the more they were ignored, actually went into convulsions from the strain, and was attended for a month by her family physician before she was able to resume the treatment. This woman was advised to stop palming, and, with her eyes open, to recall as many colours as possible, remembering each one as perfectly as possible. By thus taking the bull by the horns and consciously making the mind wander more than it did unconsciously, she became able to palm for short periods.

Some particular kinds of black objects may be found to be more easily remembered than others. Black fur, for instance, proved to be an 'optimum' (see Chapter 15) with many persons as compared to black velvet, silk, broadcloth, ink, and the letters on the test card, although it was no blacker than these other blacks. A familiar black object can often be remembered more easily by the patient than those that are less familiar. A dressmaker, for instance, was able to remember a thread of black silk when she could not remember any other black object.

When a black letter is regarded before palming, the patient will usually remember not only the blackness of the letter but the white background as well. If the

74

memory of the black is held for a few seconds, however, the background usually fades away and the whole field becomes black.

People often say, on the other hand, that they remember black perfectly when they do not. One can usually tell whether or not this is the case by noting the effect of palming upon the vision. If there is no improvement in the sight when the eyes are opened, it can be demonstrated by bringing the black closer to the patient that it has not been remembered perfectly.

Although black is, as a rule, the easiest colour to remember, for reasons explained in the next chapter, the following method sometimes succeeds when the memory of black fails. Remember a variety of colours—bright red, yellow, green, blue, purple, white especially—all in the most intense shade possible. Do not attempt to hold any of them more than a second. Keep this up for five or ten minutes. Then remember a piece of white chalk about half an inch in diameter and as white as possible. Note the colour of the background. Usually it will be a shade of black. If it is, note whether it is possible to remember anything blacker, or to see anything blacker with the eyes open. In all cases in which the white chalk is remembered perfectly, the background will be so black that it will be impossible to remember anything blacker with the eyes closed or to see anything blacker with them open.

When palming is successful, it is one of the best methods I know of for securing relaxation of all the sensory nerves, including those of sight. When perfect relaxation is gained in this way, as indicated by the ability to see a perfect black, it is completely retained when the eyes are opened, and the person's sight is permanently improved. At the same time, pain in the eyes and head and even in other parts of the body is permanently relieved. Such cases are very rare, but they do occur. With a lesser degree of relaxation much of it is lost when the eyes are opened, and what is retained is not held permanently. In other words, the greater the degree of the relaxation produced by palming, the more of it is retained when the eyes are opened and the longer it lasts. If you palm perfectly, when you open your eyes you retain all of the relaxation that you gain, and you do not lose it again. If you palm imperfectly, you retain only part of what you gain and retain it only temporarily—it may be for only a few moments. Even the smallest degree of relaxation is useful, however, for by means of it a still greater degree may be obtained.

Persons who succeed with palming from the beginning are to be congratulated, for they are always relieved very quickly. A very remarkable case of this kind was that of a man nearly seventy years of age with compound hypermetropic astigmatism and presbyopia, complicated by incipient cataract. For more than forty years he had worn glasses to improve his distant vision, and for twenty years he had worn them for reading and desk work. Because of the cloudiness of the lens of his eye he had become unable to see well enough to do his work even with glasses, and other physicians whom he had consulted had given him no hope of relief except operation when the cataract was ripe. When he found palming helped him, he asked:

'Can I do that too much.?

'No,' he was told. 'Palming is simply a means of resting your eyes, and you cannot rest them too much.'

A few days later he returned and said:

'Doctor, it was tedious, very tedious, but I did it.'

'What was tedious?' I asked.

'Palming,' he replied. 'I did it continuously for twenty hours."

'But you couldn't have kept it up for twenty hours continuously,' I said incredulously. 'You must have stopped to eat.

Then he told me that from four o'clock in the morning until twelve at night he had eaten nothing, only drinking large quantities of water, and had devoted practically all of the time to palming. It must have been tedious, as he said, but it was also worthwhile. When he looked at the test card, without glasses, he read the bottom line at twenty feet. He also read fine print at six inches and at twenty. The cloudiness of the lens had become much better, and in the centre it had entirely disappeared. Two years later there had been no relapse.

Although the majority of persons are helped by palming, a minority are unable to see black and only increase their strain by trying to get relaxation in this way. In most cases it is possible, by using some or all of the various methods outlined in this chapter, to enable a person to palm successfully; but if much difficulty is experienced, it is usually better and more expeditious to drop the method until the sight has been improved by other means. The person may then become able to see black when he palms, but some succeed in doing it until their sight has been improved.

10

Memory as an Aid to Vision

WHEN the mind is able to remember perfectly any phenomenon of the senses, it is always perfectly relaxed. The sight is normal, if the eyes are open; and when they are closed and covered so as to exclude all the light, one sees a perfectly black field—that is, nothing at all. If you can remember the ticking of a watch or an odour or a taste perfectly, your mind is perfectly at rest and you will see a perfect black when your eyes are closed and covered. If your memory of a sensation of touch could be equal to the reality, you would see nothing but black when the light was excluded from your eyes. If you were to remember a bar of music perfectly when your eyes were closed and covered, you would see nothing but black.

But in the case of any of these phenomena it is not easy to test the correctness of the memory, and the same is true of colours other than black. All other colours including white, are altered by the amount of light to which they are exposed, and are seldom seen as perfectly as it is possible for the normal eye to see them. But when the sight is normal, black is just as black in a dim light as in a bright one. It is also just as black at the distance as at the near-point, while a small area is just as black as a large one, and in fact appears blacker.

(Black is, moreover, more readily available than any other colour; there is nothing blacker than printer's ink, and that is almost ubiquitous.) By means of the memory of black, therefore, it is possible to measure accurately one's own relaxation. If the colour is remembered perfectly, one is perfectly relaxed. If it is remembered almost perfectly, one's relaxation is almost perfect. If it cannot be remembered at all, one has very little or no relaxation.

By means of simultaneous retinoscopy, these facts can be readily demonstrated. An absolutely perfect memory is very rare, so rare that it need hardly be taken into consideration; but an almost perfect memory, or what might be called normal, is attainable by everyone under certain conditions. With such a memory of black, the retinoscope shows that all errors of refraction are corrected. If the memory is less than normal, the contrary will be the case. If it fluctuates, the shadow of the retinoscope will fluctuate.

The testimony of the retinoscope is, in fact, more reliable than the statements of the patient. Patients often believe and state that they remember black perfectly, or normally, when the retinoscope indicates an error of refraction, but in such cases it can usually be demonstrated by bringing a test card to the point at which the black letters can be seen best, that the memory is not equal to the sight. The reader can easily demonstrate that the colour cannot be remembered perfectly when the eyes and mind are under a strain, by trying to remember it when making a conscious effort to see—by staring, partly closing the eyes, frowning etc.—or while trying to see all the letters of a line equally well at one time. It will be found that it either cannot be remembered at all under these conditions or is re-membered very imperfectly.

When the two eyes of a person are different, it has been found that the difference can be exactly measured by the length of time a black full stop can be remembered, while looking at a test card with both eyes open and then with the better eye closed. A person with normal vision in the right eye and half-normal vision in the left could, when looking at the test card with both eyes open, remember a full stop for twenty seconds continuously; with the better eye closed, it could be remembered for only ten seconds. A person with half-normal vision in the right eye and quarter-normal in the left could remember a full stop for twelve seconds with both eyes open and for only six seconds with the better eye closed. A third person, with normal sight in the right eye and vision of one-tenth in the left, could remember a full stop for twenty seconds with both eyes open and for only two seconds when the better eye was closed. In other words, if the right eye is better than the left, the memory is better when the right eye is open than when only the left eye is open, the difference being in exact proportion to the difference in the vision of the two eyes.

In the treatment of functional eye troubles this relationship between relaxation and memory is of great practical importance. The sensations of the eye and of the mind supply very little information as to the strain to which both are being subjected, those who strain most often suffering the least discomfort; but by means of his ability to remember black a person can always know whether he is straining or not, and is therefore able to avoid the conditions that produce strain. Whatever method of improving his sight the person is using, he is advised to carry with him constantly the memory of a small area of black, such as a full stop, so that he may recognize and avoid the conditions that produce strain. In some cases persons have been completely relieved in a very short time by this means alone. One advantage of the method is that it does not require a test card, for at any hour of the day or night, whatever the person may be doing, he can always place himself in circumstances favourable to the perfect memory of a full stop.

The condition of mind in which a black full stop can be remembered cannot be attained by any sort of effort. The memory is not the cause of the relaxation, it must be preceded by it. It is obtained only during moments of relaxation and is retained only as long as the causes of strain are avoided; but how this is accomplished cannot be fully explained, just as many other psychological phenomena cannot be completely explained. We only know that under certain conditions that might be called favourable, a degree of relaxation sufficient for the memory of a black full stop is possible, and that, by persistently seeking these conditions, a person becomes able to increase the degree of the relaxation and prolong its duration, finally becoming able to retain it under unfavourable conditions.

For most people palming provides the most favourable conditions for the memory of black. When the strain to see is lessened by the exclusion of the light, a person is usually able to remember a black object for a few seconds or longer, and this period of relaxation can be prolonged in one of two ways Either the person can open his eyes and look at a black object by central fixation at the distance at which it can be seen best,

81

and at which the eyes are therefore most relaxed, or he can shift mentally from one black object to another or from one part of a black object to another. By these means, and perhaps also through other influences that are not clearly understood, most people sooner or later become able to remember black for an indefinite length of time with their eyes closed and covered.

With the eyes open and looking at a blank surface without consciously trying to see, the unconscious strain is lessened so that the person becomes able to remember a black full stop, and all errors of refraction, as demonstrated by the retinoscope, are corrected. This result has been found to be invariable, and so long as the surface remains blank and the person does not begin to remember or imagine things seen imperfectly, the memory and the vision may be retained. But if, with the improved vision, details upon the surface begin to come out, or if the person begins to think of the test card, which he has seen imperfectly, the strain to see will return and the full stop will be lost.

When looking at a surface on which there is nothing particular to see, distance makes no difference to the memory, because a person can always look at such a surface, no matter where it is, without straining to see it. When looking to letters or other details, however, the memory is best at the point at which a person's sight is best, because at that point the eyes and mind are more relaxed than when the same letters or objects are regarded at distances at which the vision is not so good. By practising central fixation at the most favourable distances, therefore, and using any other means of improving the vision which are found to be effective the memory of the full stop may be improved, in some cases very rapidly.

If the relaxation gained under these favourable conditions is perfect, a person will be able to retain it when the mind is conscious of the impressions of sight at unfavourable distances. Such cases are, however, very rare. Usually the degree of relaxation gained is markedly imperfect, and is thus lost to a greater or lesser degree when the conditions are unfavourable, as when letters or objects are being regarded at unfavourable distances. So disturbing are the impressions of sight under these circumstances that just as soon as details begin to come out at distances at which they have not previously been seen, the patient usually loses his relaxation, and with it the memory of the full stop. In fact, the strain to see may even return before he has had time to become conscious of the image on his retina, as the following case strikingly illustrates.

A woman of fifty-five who had myopia of fifteen diopters, complicated with other conditions which made it impossible for her to see the big C at more than one foot, or to go about either in her house or on the street without an attendant, became able, when she looked at a green wall without trying to see it, to remember a perfectly black full stop and to see a small area of the wallpaper at the distance as well as she could at the near-point. When she had come close to the wall she was asked to put her hand on the doorknob, which she did without hesitation. 'But I don't see the knob,' she hastened to explain. As a matter of fact she had seen it long enough to put her hand on it, but as soon as the idea of seeing it was suggested to her she lost the memory of the full stop, and with it her improved vision, and when she again tried to find the knob she could not do so.

When a full stop is remembered perfectly while a letter on a test card is being regarded, the letter improves, with or without consciousness; it is impossible to strain and relax at the same time, and if one relaxes sufficiently to remember the full stop, one must also relax sufficiently to see the letter, consciously or unconsciously. Letters on either side of the one regarded, or on the lines above and below it, also improve. When a person is conscious of seeing the letters this is very distracting and usually causes him, at first, to forget the full stop. With some people, as already noted, the strain may return even before the letters are consciously recognized.

Thus people find themselves on the horns of a dilemma. The relaxation indicated by the memory of a full stop improves their sight, and the things they see with this improved vision cause them to lose their relaxation and their memory. It is very remarkable to me how the difficulty is ever overcome, but some people are able to do it in five minutes or half an hour. With others the process is long and tedious.

There are various ways to deal with this situation. One is to remember the full stop while looking a little to one side of the test card, say a foot or more, then to look a little nearer to it, and finally to look between the lines. In this way a person may become able to see the letters in the eccentric field without losing the full stop, and when he can do this he may become able to go a step farther and look directly at a letter without losing control of his memory. If he cannot do it, he can look at only one part of a letter—usually the bottom—or see or imagine the full stop as part of the letter, while noting that the rest of the letter is less black and less distinct than the part directly regarded. When he can do this he becomes able to remember the full stop better than when the letter is seen all alike. If the letter is seen all alike, the perfect memory of the full stop is always lost.

The next step is to note whether the bottom of the letter is straight, curved, or open, without losing the full stop on the bottom. When a person can do this he can try to do the same with the sides and top of the letter, still holding the full stop on the bottom. Usually when the parts can be observed separately in this way, the whole letter can be seen without losing the memory of the full stop; but it occasionally happens that this is not the case, and further practice is needed before a person can become conscious of all sides of the letter at once without losing the full stop. This may require moments, hours, days, or months. In one case the following method succeeded.

A man with fifteen diopters of myopia was so much disturbed by what he saw when his vision had been improved by the memory of a full stop that he was directed to look away from the test card, or whatever object he was regarding. He found the letters or other details coming out. For about a week he went around persistently dodging his improved sight. As his memory improved it became more and more difficult for him to do this, and at the end of the week it was impossible. When he looked at the bottom line at a distance of twenty feet he remembered the full stop perfectly, and when asked if he could see the letters he replied,

'I cannot help seeing them.'

Some people retard their recovery by decorating the scenery with full stops as they go about during the day,

85

instead of simply remembering a full stop in their minds. This does them no good, but is, on the contrary, a cause of strain. The full stop can be imagined perfectly and with benefit as forming part of a black letter on the test card, because this merely means imagining that one sees one part of the black letter best; but it cannot be imagined perfectly on any surface which is not black and to attempt to imagine it on any other surface defeats the end in view.

The smaller the area of black which a person is able to remember, the greater is the degree of relaxation indicated, but some people find it easier at first to remember a somewhat larger area, such as one of the letters on a test card with one part blacker than the rest. They may begin with the big C, then proceed to the smaller letters, and finally get to a full stop. It is then found that this small area is remembered more easily than the larger ones, and that its black is more intense. Instead of a full stop, some people find it easier to remember a colon, with one full stop blacker than the other, or a collection of full stops, with one blacker than all the others, or the dot over a small I or J. Others, again, prefer a comma to a full stop.

In the beginning most people find it helpful to shift consciously from one of these black areas to another, or from one part of such an area to another, and to realize the swing, or pulsation produced by such shifting (see Chapter 12). But when the memory becomes perfect, one object may be held continuously without conscious shifting, while the swing is realized only when attention is directed to the matter.

Although black is usually the best colour to remember, some people are bored or depressed by it and prefer to remember white or some other colour. A familiar object, or one with pleasant associations, is often easier to remember than one which has no particular interest. One woman's sight was corrected by the memory of a yellow buttercup, and another was able to remember the opal of her ring when she could not remember a full stop. Whatever the person finds easiest to remember is the best to remember, because the memory can never be perfect unless it is easy.

When the memory of the full stop becomes habitual, it is not only not a burden but also a great help to other mental processes. The mind, when it remembers one thing better than all other things, possesses central fixation, and its efficiency is thereby increased just as the efficiency of the eye is increased by central fixation. In other words, the mind attains its greatest efficiency when it is at rest, and it is never at rest unless one thing is remembered better than all other things. When the mind is in such a condition that a full stop is remembered perfectly, the memory of other things is improved.

A high-school girl reports that when she was unable to remember the answer to a question in an examination, she remembered the full stop and the answer came to her. When I cannot remember the name of a patient, I remember a full stop—and behold, I have it! A musician who had perfect sight and could remember a full stop perfectly had a perfect memory for music, but a musician with imperfect sight who could not remember a full stop could play nothing without his notes, only gaining that power when his sight and visual memory had become normal. In some exceptional cases, the strain to see letters on a test card has been so terrific that people have said that while they were looking at them they could remember neither the full stop nor their own names.

A person may measure the accuracy of his memory of the full stop not only by comparing it with the sight but by the following tests:

When the memory of the full stop is perfect, it is instantaneous. If a few seconds or longer are necessary to obtain that memory, it is never perfect.

A perfect memory is not only instantaneous but also continuous.

When the full stop is remembered perfectly, normal sight comes instantaneously. If good vision is obtained only after a second or two, it can always be demonstrated that the memory of the full stop is imperfect and the sight also.

The memory of a full stop is a test of relaxation. It is the evidence by which a person knows that his eyes and mind are at rest. It may be compared to the steam gauge of an engine, which has nothing to do with the machinery, but is of great importance in giving information as to the ability of the mechanism to do its work. When the full stop is black, one knows that the engine of the eye is in good working order. When the full stop fades or is lost, one knows that the engine is out of order, until a cure is effected. Then one does not need a full stop, or any other aid to vision, just as the engineer does not need a steam gauge when the engine is going properly.

A man who had gained telescopic and microscopic vision by the methods presented in this book said, in answer to an inquiry from someone interested in investigating the treatment of errors of refraction without glasses, that he not only had done nothing to prevent a relapse but had even forgotten how he was cured. The reply was unsatisfactory to the inquirer; but it is quoted to illustrate the fact that when a person's sight is corrected he does not need to do anything consciously in order to keep it so, although the treatment can always be continued with benefit since even supernormal vision can be improved.

11

Imagination as an Aid to Vision

WE see very largely with the mind, and only partly
with the eyes. The phenomena of vision depend upon
the mind's interpretation of the impression upon the
retina. What we see is not that impression but our own
interpretation of it. Our impressions of size, colour,
form and location can be shown to depend upon the
interpretation by the mind of the retinal picture. The
moon looks smaller at the zenith than it does at the
horizon, though the optical angle is the same and the
impression on the retina may be the same, because at the
horizon the mind unconsciously compares the picture
with the pictures of surrounding objects, while at the
zenith there is nothing to compare it with. The figure of
a man on a high building, or on the topmast of a ship,
looks small to the landsman, but to the sailor it
appears to be of ordinary size, because he is accustomed
to seeing the human figure in such positions.

Persons with normal vision use their memory, or
imagination, as an aid to sight; and when the sight is
imperfect it can be demonstrated, not only that the eye
itself is at fault, but that the memory and imagination
are impaired so that the mind adds imperfections to
the imperfect retinal image. No two persons with
normal sight will get the same visual impressions from

the same object, for their interpretations of the retinal picture will differ as much as their individualities differ, and when the sight is imperfect the interpretation is far more variable. It reflects, in fact, the loss of mental control, which is responsible for the error of refraction. When the eye is out of focus, in short, the mind is also out of focus.

According to the accepted view, most of the abnormalities of vision produced when there is an error of refraction in the eye are sufficiently accounted for by the existence of that error. Some are supposed to be due to diseases of the brain or retina. Multiple images are attributed to astigmatism, though only two can be legitimately accounted for in this way (since no one has more than two eyes). Some persons state that they see half a dozen or more, and many persons with astigmatism do not see any. It can easily be demonstrated, however, that the inaccuracy of the focus accounts for only a small part of these results, and since they can all be corrected in a few seconds through the correction, by relaxation, of the error of refraction, it is evident that they cannot be due to any organic disease.

If we compare the picture on the glass screen of the camera when the camera is out of focus with the visual impressions of the mind when the eye is out of focus, there will be found a great difference between them. When the camera is out of focus it turns black into grey and blurs the outlines of the picture, but it produces these results uniformly and constantly. On the screen of the camera an imperfect picture of a black letter would be equally imperfect in all parts, and the same adjustment of the focus would always produce the same picture. But when the eye is out of focus the

91

imperfect picture which a person imagines that he sees is always changing, whether the focus changes or not. There will be more grey on one part than on another and both the shade and the position of the grey may vary within wide limits in a very short space of time. One part of a letter may appear grey and the rest black. Certain outlines may be seen better than others, the vertical lines, perhaps, appearing black and the diagonal grey, and vice versa. Again, the black may be changed into brown, yellow, green, or even red, transmutations which are impossible in the camera. Or there may be spots of colour, or of black, on the grey or on the white openings. There may also be spots of white, or of colour, on the black.

When the camera is out of focus the picture which it produces of any object is always slightly larger than the image produced when the focus is correct, but when the eye is out of focus the picture which the mind sees may be either larger or smaller than it would normally be. To one person the big C at ten feet appeared smaller than at either twenty feet or four inches. To some it appears larger than it actually is at twenty feet, and to others it seems smaller.

When the human eye is out of focus the form of the objects regarded by the patient frequently appears to be distorted, while their location may also appear to change. The image may be doubled, tripled, or still further multiplied, and while one object or part of an object may be multiplied, other objects or parts of objects in the field of vision may remain single. The location of these multiple images is at some times constant and at others subject to continual change. Nothing like this could happen when the camera is out of focus.

If two cameras are out of focus of the same degree they will take two imperfect pictures exactly alike. If two eyes are out of focus to the same degree, similar impressions will be made upon the retina of each, but the impressions made upon the mind may be totally unlike, whether the eyes belong to the same person or to different persons. If the normal eye looks at an object through glasses that change its refraction, the greyness and blurring produced are uniform and constant, but when the eye has an error of refraction equivalent to that produced by the glasses, these phenomena are nonuniform and variable.

It is fundamental that a person should understand that these aberrations of vision—which are treated more fully in a later chapter—are illusions, and are not due to a fault of the eyes. When one knows that a thing is an illusion, he is less likely to see it again. When he becomes convinced that what he sees is imaginary, it helps to bring the imagination under control, and since a perfect imagination is impossible without perfect relaxation, a perfect imagination not only corrects the false interpretation of the retinal image but corrects the error of refraction.

Imagination is closely allied to memory, although distinct from it. Imagination depends upon the memory, because a thing can be imagined only as well as it can be remembered. You cannot imagine a sunset unless you have seen one. If you attempt to imagine a blue sun, which you have never seen, you will become myopic, as indicated by simultaneous retinoscopy. Neither imagination nor memory can be perfect unless the mind is perfectly relaxed. Therefore, when the imagination and memory are perfect, the sight is perfect (unless the eye had some physical defect). Imagination, memory and sight are, in fact, coincident. When one is perfect, all are perfect, and when one is imperfect, all are imperfect. If you imagine a letter perfectly, you will see that the letter and other letters in its neighbourhood will come out more distinctly, because it is impossible for you to relax and imagine you see a perfect letter and at the same time strain and actually see an imperfect one. If you imagine a perfect full stop on the bottom of a letter, you will see the letter perfectly, because you cannot take the mental picture of a perfect full stop and put it on an imperfect letter. It is possible, however, as pointed out in the preceding chapter, for sight to be unconscious. In some cases people may magine the full stop perfectly, as demonstrated by the retinoscope, without being conscious of seeing the letter, and it is often some time before they are able to be conscious of it without losing the full stop.

When a person is willing to believe that the letters can be imagined, and is content to imagine without trying to see, or to compare what he sees with what he imagines, which always brings back the strain, very remarkable results are sometimes obtained by the aid of the imagination. Some people at once become able to read all the letters on the bottom line of the test card after they become able to imagine that they see one letter perfectly black and distinct. The majority, however, are so distracted by what they see when their vision has been improved by their imagination that they lose the latter. It is one thing to be able to imagine perfect sight of a letter, and another to be able to see the letter and other letters without losing control of the imagination.

In myopia the following method is often successful. First look at a letter at the point at which it is seen best. Then close the eyes and remember it. Repeat until the memory is almost as good as the sight at the near-point. With the test card at a distance of twenty feet, look at a blank surface a foot or more to one side of it, and again remember the letter. Do the same at six inches and at three inches. At the last point note the appearance of the letters on the card—that is, in the eccentric field. If the memory is still perfect, they will appear to be a dim black, not grey, and those nearest the point of fixation will appear blacker than those further away. Gradually reduce the distance between the point of fixation and the letter until you can look straight at it and imagine that it is seen as well as it is remembered. Occasionally it is well during this practice to close and cover the eyes and remember the letter, or a full stop, perfectly black. The rest and mental control gained in this way are a help in gaining control when one looks at the test card.

People who succeed with this method are not conscious, while imagining a perfect letter, of seeing at the same time an imperfect one, and are not distracted when their vision is improved by their imagination. Many people can remember perfectly with their eyes closed, or when they are looking at a place where they cannot see the letter, but just as soon as they look at it they begin to strain and lose control of their memory. Therefore, as the imagination depends upon the memory, they cannot imagine that they see the letter. In such cases it has been my custom to proceed somewhat in the manner described in the preceding chapter. I begin by saying:

'Can you imagine a black full stop on the bottom of

this letter, and at the same time, while imagining the full stop perfectly, are you able to imagine that you see the letter?'

Sometimes they are able to do this, but usually they are not. In that case they are asked to imagine part of the letter, usually the bottom. When they can imagine this part straight, curved or open, as the case may be, they can imagine the sides and top, while still holding the full stop on the bottom. But even after they have done this, they may still be unable to imagine the whole letter without losing the full stop. I may have to coax them along by bringing the card up a little closer, then moving it farther away; for when looking at a surface where there is anything to see, the imagination improves in proportion as one approaches the point where the sight is best, since at that point the eyes are most relaxed. When there is nothing particular to see, the distance makes no difference, since no effort is being made to see.

To encourage people to imagine they see the letter, it seems helpful to keep saying to them over and over again,

'Of course you do not see the letter. I am not asking you to see it. I am just asking you to *imagine* that you see it perfectly black and perfectly distinct.'

When people become able to see a known letter by the aid of their imagination, they become able to apply the same method to an unknown letter; for just as soon as any part of a letter, such as an area equal to a full stop, can be imagined to be perfectly black, the whole letter is seen to be black, although at first the visual perception of this fact may not last long enough for a person to become conscious of it.

In trying to distinguish unknown letters, a person discovers that it is impossible to imagine perfectly unless one imagines the truth; for if a letter, or any part of a letter, is imagined to be other than it is, the mental picture is foggy and inconstant, just like a letter which is seen imperfectly.

The ways in which the imagination can be interfered with are very numerous. There is one way of imagining perfectly, and an infinite number of ways of imagining imperfectly. The right way is easy. The mental picture of the thing imagined comes as quickly as thought, and can be held more or less continuously. The wrong way is difficult. The picture comes slowly, and is both variable and discontinuous.

This can be demonstrated by first imagining or remembering a black letter as perfectly as possible with the eyes closed, and then imagining the same letter imperfectly. The first can usually be done easily, but it will be found very difficult to imagine that a black letter with clear outlines is grey with fuzzy edges and clouded openings, and impossible to form a mental picture of it that will remain constant for an appreciable length of time. The letter will vary in colour, shape and location in the visual field, percisely as a letter does when it is seen imperfectly, and just as the strain of imperfect sight produces discomfort and pain, the effort to imagine imperfectly will sometimes produce pain. The more nearly perfect the central picture of the letter, on the contrary, the more easily and quickly it comes and the more constant it is.

Some very dramatic improvements have been effected by means of the imagination. One man. a physician who had worn glasses for forty years and without them could not see the big C at twenty feet, was relieved in fifteen minutes simply by imagining that he saw the letters black. When asked to describe the big C with unaided vision, he said that it looked grey to him and that the opening was obscured by a grey cloud to such an extent that he had to guess that it had an opening. He was told that the letter was black, perfectly black, and that the opening was perfectly white, with no grey cloud, and the card was brought close to him so that he could see that this was so. When he again looked at the letter at the distance, he remembered its blackness so vividly that he was able to imagine that he saw it just as black as he had seen it at the near-point, with the opening perfectly white: therefore he saw the letter on the card perfectly black and distinct. In the same way he became able to read the seventy line, and so he went down the card, until in about five minutes he could read at twenty feet the line which the normal eye is supposed to read at ten feet. Next, diamond type was given to him to read. The letters appeared grey to him, and he could not read them. His attention was called to the fact that the letters were really black, and immediately he imagined that he saw them black and became able to read them at ten inches.

The explanation of this remarkable occurrence is simply relaxation. All the nerves of the doctor's body were relaxed when he imagined that he saw the letters black, and when he became conscious of seeing the letters on the card he still retained control of his imagination. Thus he did not begin to strain again, and actually saw the letters as black as he imagined them.

The doctor had no relapse, and he continued to improve. About a year later I visited him in his office and asked him how he was getting on. He replied that his sight was perfect, both for distance and for the near-point. He could see the automobiles on the other side of the Hudson River and the people in them, and he could read the names of boats on the river which other people could make out only with a telescope. At the same time he had no difficulty in reading the newspapers, and to prove the latter part of this statement he picked up a newspaper and read a few sentences aloud. I was astonished, and asked him how he did it.

'I did what you told me to do,' he said.

'What did I tell you to do?' I asked.

'You told me to read the test card every day, which I have done, and to read fine print every day in a dim light, which I have also done.

Another man who had a high degree of myopia complicated with atrophy of the optic nerve, and who had been discouraged by many physicians, was benefitted to such an extent and so rapidly by the aid of his imagination that one day in my office he lost control of himself completely. Raising a test card which he held in his hand, he threw it across the room.

'It is too good to be true,' he exclaimed 'I cannot believe it. The possibility of being cured and the fear of disappointment are more than I can stand.'

He was calmed down with some difficulty and encouraged to continue. Later he was able to read the small letters on the test card with normal vision. He was then given fine print to read. When he looked at the diamond type, he at once said that it was impossible for him to read it. However, he was told to follow the same procedure that had helped his distant sight. That is, he was to imagine a full stop on one part of the small letters while holding the type at six inches. After testing his memory of the full stop a number of times, he became able to imagine that he saw a full

99

stop perfectly black on one of the small letters. Then he became nervous again, and when asked what the trouble was, he said:

'I am beginning to read the fine print, and I am so overwhelmed that I lose my self-control.'

In another case, that of a woman with high myopia complicated with incipient cataract, the vision improved in a few days from 3/200 to 20/50. Instead of going gradually down the card, a jump was made from the fifty line to the ten line. The card was brought up close to her and she was asked to look at the letter O at three inches, the distance at which she saw it best, and to imagine that she saw a full stop on the bottom of it, and that the bottom was the blackest part. When she was able to do this at the near-point, the distance was gradually increased until she became able to see the O at three feet. Then I placed the card at ten feet and she exclaimed:

'Oh, Doctor, it is impossible! The letter is too small. Let me try a larger one first.'

Nevertheless, in fifteen minutes she became able to read the small O on the ten line at twenty feet.

12

Shifting and Swinging

WHEN the eye with normal vision regards a letter either at the near-point or at the distance, the letter may appear to pulsate, or to move in various directions, from side to side, up and down, or obliquely. When it looks from one letter to another on a test card, or from one side of a letter to another, not only the letter but the whole line of letters and the whole card may appear to move from side to side. This apparent movement is due to the shifting of the eye, and is always in a direction contrary to its movement.

If one looks at the top of a letter, the letter is below the line of vision and therefore appears to move downward. If one looks at the bottom, the letter is above the line of vision and appears to move upward. If one looks to the left to the letter, it is to the right to the line of vision and appears to move to the right. If one looks to the right, it is to the left of the line of vision and appears to move to the left.

Persons with normal vision are rarely conscious of this illusion and may have difficulty in demonstrating it, but in every case that has come under my observation they have always become able, in a longer or a shorter time, to do so. When the sight is imperfect, the letters may remain stationary or even move in the same direction as the eye.

It is impossible for the eye to fix a point longer than a fraction of a second. If it tries to do so, it begins to strain and the vision is lowered. This can readily be demonstrated by trying to hold one part of a letter for an appreciable length of time. No matter how good the sight, it will begin to blur, or even disappear, very quickly, and sometimes the effort to hold it will produce pain. In the case of a few exceptional people, a point may appear to be held for a considerable length of time and the subjects themselves may think that they are holding it, but this is only because the eye shifts unconsciously, the movements being so rapid that objects seem to be seen all alike simultaneously.

The shifting of the eye with normal vision is usually not conspicuous, but by direct examination with the ophthalmoscope it can always be demonstrated. If one eye is examined with this instrument while the other is regarding a small area straight ahead, the eye being examined, which follows the movements of the other, is seen to move in various directions, from side to side and up and down in an orbit which is usually variable. If the vision is normal these movements are extremely rapid and are not accompanied by any appearance of effort. The shifting of the eye with imperfect sight, on the contrary, is slower, its excursions are wider, and the movements are jerky and made with apparent effort.

It can also be demonstrated that the eye is capable of shifting with a rapidity which the ophthalmoscope cannot measure. The normal eye can read fourteen letters on the bottom line of a Snellen test card, at a distance of ten or fifteen feet, in a dim light, so rapidly that they seem to be seen all at once. Yet it can be shown that in order to recognize the letters under these conditions it is necessary to make about four shifts to each letter. At the near-point, even though one part of the letter is seen best, the rest may be seen well enough to be recognized; but at the distance it is impossible to recognize the letters unless one shifts from the top to the bottom and from side to side. One must also shift from one letter to another, making about seventy shifts in a fraction of a second.

A line of small letters on the Snellen test card may be less than a foot long by a quarter of an inch in height, and if it requires seventy shifts to a fraction of a second to see it apparently all at once, it must require many thousands of shifts to see an area, the size of a motion picture screen, with all its detail of people, animals, houses, or trees. To see sixteen such areas to a second, as we do in viewing a motion picture, must require a rapidity of shifting that can scarcely be realized.

Not only are the human eye and mind capable of this rapidity of action, and that without effort or strain, but it is only when the eye is able to shift this rapidly that eye and mind are at rest, and the efficiency of both at their maximum. It is true that every motion of the eye produces an error of refraction, but when the movement is short this is very slight. Usually the shifts are so rapid that the error does not last long enough to be detected by the retinoscope, its existence being demonstrable only by reducing the rapidity of the movements to less than four or five a second. The period during which the eye is at rest is much longer than that during which an error of refraction is produced. Hence, when the eye shifts normally no error of refraction is manifest. The more rapid the unconscious shifting of the eye, the better the vision; but if one tries to be conscious of a too rapid shift, a strain will be produced.

Normal sight is impossible without continual shifting, and such shifting is a striking illustration of the mental control necessary for normal vision. It requires perfect mental control to think of thousands of things in a fraction of a second, and each point of fixation has to be thought of separately, because it is impossible to think of two things, or of two parts of one thing, perfectly at the same time. The eye with imperfect sight tries to accomplish the impossible by looking fixedly at one point for an appreciable length of time—that is, by staring. When it looks at a strange letter and does not see it, it keeps on looking at it in an effort to see it better. Such efforts always fail, and are an important factor in the production of imperfect sight.

One of the best methods of improving the sight, we now find, is to imitate consciously the unconscious shifting of normal vision and to realize the apparent motion produced by such shifting. Whether one has imperfect or normal sight, conscious shifting and swinging are a great help and advantage to the eye: not only imperfect sight but also normal sight may be improved in this way. When the sight is imperfect, shifting, if done properly, rests the eye as much as palming, and always lessens or corrects the error of refraction.

The eye with normal sight never attempts to hold a point more than a fraction of a second, and when it shifts, as explained in Chapter 8, it always sees the previous point of fixation worse. When it ceases to shift rapidly and to see the point shifted from worse, the sight ceases to be normal, the swing being either prevented or lengthened, or occasionally reversed. These facts are the keynote of treatment by shifting.

In order to see the previous point of fixation worse, the eye with imperfect sight has to look farther away from it than does the eye with normal sight. If the eye shifts only a quarter of an inch, for instance, it may see the previous point of fixation as well as or better than before, and instead of being rested by such a shift, its strain will be increased, there will be no swing, and the vision will be lowered. At a couple of inches it may be able to let go of the first point, and if neither point is held more than a fraction of a second, it will be rested by such a shift and the illusion of swinging may be produced. The shorter the shift, the greater the benefit, but even a very long shift—as much as three feet or more—is a help to those who cannot accomplish a shorter one.

When a person is capable of a short shift, on the other hand, the long shift lowers the vision. The swing is an evidence that the shifting is being done properly, and when it occurs the vision is always improved. It is possible to shift without improvement, but it is impossible to produce the illusion of a swing without improvement; when this can be done with a long shift, the movement can gradually be shortened until a person can shift from the top to the bottom of the smallest letters, on a test card or elsewhere, and maintain the swing. Later he may become able to be conscious of the swinging of the letters without conscious shifting.

No matter how imperfect the sight, it is always possible to shift and produce a swing, so long as the previous point of fixation is seen worse. Even diplopia and polyopia (double and multiple vision, respectively) do not prevent swinging with some improvement of vision. Usually the eye with imperfect vision is able to shift from one side of the card to the other, or from a point above the card to a point below it, and observe that in the first case the card appears to move from side to side while in the second it appears to move up and down.

When people are suffering from high degrees of eccentric fixation, it may be necessary, in order to see worse when they shift, to use some of the methods described in Chapter 8. Usually, however, people who cannot see worse when they shift at the distance can do it readily at the near-point, as the sight is best at that point, not only in myopia but often in hypermetropia as well. When the swing can be produced at the near-point, the distance can be gradually increased until the same thing can be done at twenty feet.

After resting the eyes by closing or palming, shifting and swinging are often more successful. By this method of alternately resting the eyes and then shifting, persons with very imperfect sight have sometimes obtained a temporary or permanent relief in a few weeks.

Shifting may be done slowly or rapidly, according to the state of the vision. At the beginning a person will be likely to strain if he shifts too rapidly, and then the point shifted from will not be seen worse and there will be no swing. As improvement is made, the speed can be increased. It is usually impossible, however, to realize the swing if the shifting is more rapid than two or three times a second.

A mental picture of a letter can, as a rule, be made to swing precisely as can a letter on the test card. There is the occasional person with whom the opposite is true, but for most people the mental swing is easier at first than visual swinging. When they become able to swing in this way, it becomes easier for them to swing the letters on the test card. By alternating mental with visual swinging and shifting, rapid progress is sometimes made. As relaxation becomes more perfect, the mental swing can be shortened until it becomes possible to conceive and swing a letter the size of a full stop in a newspaper. This is easier, when it can be done, than swinging a larger letter, and many people have derived great benefit from it.

All persons, no matter how great their error of refraction, correct it partially or completely (as demonstrated by the retinoscope) for at least a fraction of a second when they shift and swing successfully. This time may be so short that a person is not conscious of improved vision, but it is possible for him to imagine it, and then it becomes easier to maintain the relaxation long enough to be conscious of the improved sight. For instance, after looking away from the card a person may look back to the big C, and for a fraction of a second the error of refraction may be lessened or corrected, as demonstrated by the retinoscope. Yet he may not be conscious of improved vision. By imagining that C is seen better, however, the amount of relaxation may be sufficiently prolonged to be realized.

When swinging, either mental or visual, is successful, a person may become conscious of a feeling of relaxation which is manifested as a sensation of universal swinging. This sensation communicates itself to any object of which a person is conscious. The motion may be imagined in any part of the body to which the attention is directed. It may be communicated to the chair in which a person is sitting, or to any object in the room, or elsewhere, which is remembered. The

107

building, the city, the whole world may appear to be swinging. When a person becomes conscious of this universal swinging he loses the memory of the object with which it started, but so long as he is able to maintain the movement in a direction contrary to the original movement of the eyes, or the movement imagined by the mind, relaxation is maintained. If the direction is changed, however, strain results. To imagine the universal swing with the eyes closed is easy, and some people soon become able to do it with the eyes open. Later the feeling of relaxation which accompanies the swing may be realized without consciousness of the latter, but the swing can always be produced when a person thinks of it.

There is only one cause of failure to produce a swing, and that is strain. Some people try to make the letters swing by effort. Such efforts always fail. The eyes and mind do not swing the letters, they swing of themselves. The eye can shift voluntarily. This is a muscular act resulting from a motor impulse. But the swing comes of its own accord when the shifting is normal. It does not produce relaxation, but is an evidence of it; while of no value in itself, it is, like the full stop, very valuable as an indication that relaxation is being maintained.

The following methods of shifting have been found useful in various cases:

No. 1

(a) Look at a letter on a test card.

(b) Shift to a letter on the same line far enough away so that the first is seen worse.

(c) Look back at the first and see the second worse.

(d) Look at the letters alternately for a few seconds, seeing worse the one not regarded.

When successful, both letters improve and appear to move from side to side in a direction opposite to the movement of the eye.

No. 2

(a) Look at a large letter.

(b) Look at a smaller one a long distance away from it. The large one is then seen worse.

(c) Look back and see it better.

(d) Repeat half a dozen times.

When successful, both letters improve, and the card appears to move up and down.

No. 3

Shifting by the methods above enables a person to see one letter on a line better than the other letters, and, usually, to distinguish it in flashes. In order to see the letter continuously it is necessary to be able to shift from the top to the bottom, or from the bottom to the top, seeing worse the part not directly regarded, and producing the illusion of a vertical swing.

(a) Look at a point far enough above the top of the letter to see the bottom, or the whole letter, worse.

(b) Look at a point far enough below the bottom to see the top, or the whole letter, worse.

(c) Repeat half a dozen times.

If successful, the letter will appear to move up and down, and the vision will improve. The shift can then be shortened until it becomes possible to shift between the top and the bottom of the letter and maintain the swing. The letter is now seen continuously. If the method fails, rest the eyes, palm, and try again.

One may also practice by shifting from one side of the letter to a point beyond the other side, or from one corner to a point beyond the other corner.

No. 4

(a) Look at a letter at the distance at which it is seen best. In myopia this will be at the near-point, a foot or less from the face. Shift from the top to the bottom until able to see each worse alternately, when the letter will appear blacker than before and an illusion of swinging will be produced.

(b) Now close the eyes and shift from the top to the bottom of the letter mentally.

(c) Regard a blank wall with the eyes open and repeat (b). Compare the ability to shift and swing mentally with the ability to do the same visually at the near-point.

(d) Then regard the letter at the distance and shift from top to the bottom. If successful, the letter will improve and an illusion of swinging will be produced.

No. 5

Some people, particularly children, are able to see better when someone else points to the letters. In other cases this is a distraction. When the pointing method is found successful one can proceed as follows:

(a) Have someone place the tip of his finger three or four inches below the letter. Let the person taking the treatment regard the letter and shift to the tip of the finger, seeing the letter worse.

(b) Reduce the distance between the finger and the letter, first to two or three inches, then to one or two, and finally to half an inch, proceeding each time as in (a).

If successful, the person will become able to look from the top to the bottom of the letter, seeing each worse alternately and producing the illusion of swinging. It will then be possible to see the letter continuously.

No. 6

When the vision is imperfect it often happens that when a person looks at a small letter, some of the large letters on the upper lines, or the big C at the top, look blacker than the letter looked at. This makes it impossible to see the smaller letters perfectly. To correct this eccentric fixation, regard the letter which is seen best and shift to the smaller letter. If you are successful, the small letter, after a few moments, will appear blacker than the larger one. If not successful after a few trials rest the eyes by closing and palming, and try again. One may also shift from the large letter to a point some distance below the small letter, gradually approaching the latter as the vision improves.

No. 7

Shifting from a card at three or five feet to one at ten or twenty feet often proves helpful, as the unconscious memory of the letter seen at the near-point helps to bring out the one at the distance.

Different people will find these various methods of shifting more or less satisfactory. If any method does not succeed, it should be abandoned after one or two trials and something else tried. It is a mistake to continue the practice of any method which does not yield prompt results. The cause of the failure is strain, and it does no good to continue the strain.

When it is not possible to practice with a test card, other objects may be utilized. One can shift, for instance, from one window of a distant building to another, from one part of a window to another part of the same window, from one car to another, or from one part of a car to another part, producing, in each case, the illusion that the objects are moving in a direction contrary to the movement of the eye. When talking to people, one can shift from one person to another or from one part of the face to another part. When reading a book or a newspaper, one can shift consciously from one word or letter to another, or from one part of a letter to another.

Shifting and swinging, as they give a person something definite to do, are often more successful than other methods of obtaining relaxation, and in some cases remarkable results have been obtained simply by showing a person that staring lowers the vision and shifting improves it. One patient of mine, a girl of sixteen with progressive myopia, obtained very prompt relief by shifting. She came to the office wearing a pair of glasses tinted a pale yellow, with shades at the sides; in spite of this protection she was so annoyed by the light that her eyes were almost closed and she had great difficulty in finding her way about the room. Her vision without glasses was 3/200. All reading had been forbidden, playing the piano from the notes was not

112

allowed, and she had been obliged to give up the idea of going to college.

Her sensitiveness to light was relieved in a few minutes by a sun treatment (described in Chapter 24) on her closed eyes. She was then seated before a test card and directed to look away from it, rest her eyes, and then look at the big C. For a fraction of a second her vision was improved, and by frequent demonstrations she was made to realize that any effort to see the letters always lowered the vision. By alternately looking away and then looking back at the letters for a fraction of a second, her vision improved so rapidly that in the course of half an hour it was almost normal for the distance.

Then she was given diamond type to read. The attempt to read it at once brought on severe pain. She was directed to proceed as she had in reading the test card, and in a few minutes, by alternately looking away and then looking at the first letter of each word in turn, she became able to read without fatigue, discomfort, or pain. She left the office without her glasses, and was able to see her way without difficulty. Other patients have been benefitted as promptly by this simple method.

13

The Illusions of Sight

PERSONS with imperfect sight always have illusions of vision; so do persons with normal sight. But while the illusions of normal sight are an evidence of relaxation, the illusions of imperfect sight are an evidence of strain. Some persons with errors of refraction have few illusions, others have many, because the strain which causes the error of refraction is not the same strain that is responsible for the illusions.

The illusions of imperfect sight may relate to the colour, size, location, and form of the objects regarded. They may include appearances of things that have no existence at all, and various other curious and interesting manifestations.

Illusions of Colour

When a person sees a black letter and believes it to be grey, yellow, brown, blue, or green, he is suffering from an illusion of colour. This phenomenon differs from colour-blindness. The colour-blind person is unable to differentiate between different colours, usually blue and green, and his inability to do so is constant. The person suffering from an illusion of colour does not see the false colours constantly or uniformly. When he looks at a test card the black letters may appear to him to be grey at one time, but at another moment they may appear to be a shade of yellow, blue, or brown. Some people always see the black letters red; to others, they appear red only occasionally. Although the letters are all of the same colour, some may see the large letters black and the small ones yellow or blue. Usually the large letters are seen darker than the small ones, whatever colour they appear to be. Often different colours appear in the same letter, part of it seeming to be black, perhaps, and the rest grey or some other colour. Spots of black, or of colour, may appear on the white, and spots of white, or of colour, on the black.

Illusions of Size

Large letters may appear small, or small letters large. One letter may appear to be of normal size, while another of the same size and at the same distance may appear larger or smaller than normal. A letter may appear to be of normal size at the near-point and at the distance, but only half that size at the middle distance. When a person can judge the size of a letter correctly at all distances up to twenty feet, his vision is normal. If the size appears different to him at different distances, he is suffering from an illusion of size. At great distances the judgment of size is always imperfect, because the sight at such distances is imperfect, even though perfect at ordinary distances. The stars appear to be dots, because the eye does not possess perfect vision for objects at such distances. A candle seen half a mile away appears smaller than at the near-point, but seen through a telescope giving perfect vision at that distance, it will be the same as at the near-point. With improved vision the ability to judge size improves.

The correction of an error of refraction by glasses seldom enables a person to judge size as correctly as the normal eye can, and the ability to do this may differ very greatly in persons having the same error of refraction. A person with ten diopters of myopia corrected by glasses may (rarely) be able to judge the sizes of objects correctly. Another person with the same degree of myopia and the same glasses may see things only one-half or one-third their normal size. This indicates that errors of refraction have very little to do with incorrect perceptions of size.

Illusions of Form

Round letters may appear square or triangular; straight letters may appear curved; letters of regular form may appear very irregular; a round letter may appear to have a checker-board or a cross in the centre. In short, an infinite variety of changing forms may be seen. Illumination, distance and environment are all factors in this form of imperfect sight. Many persons can see the form of a letter correctly when other letters are covered, but when the other letters are visible they cannot see it. The indication of the position of a letter by a pointer helps some people to see it. Others are so disturbed by the pointer that they cannot see the letter so well.

Illusions of Number

Multiple images are frequently seen by persons with imperfect sight, either with both eyes together, with each eye separately, or with only one eye. The manner in which these multiple images make their appearance is sometimes very curious. For instance, a patient with presbyopia read the word HAS normally with both eyes. The word PHONES he read correctly with the left eye, but when he read it with the right eye he saw the letter P double, the imaginary image being a little distance to the left of the real one. The left eye, while it had normal vision for the word PHONES, multiplied the shaft of a pin when this object was in a vertical position, although the head remained single, and multiplied the head when the position was changed to the horizontal, the shaft then remaining single. When the point of the pin was placed below a very small letter, the point was sometimes doubled while the letter remained single.

No error of refraction can account for these phenomena. They are tricks of the mind only. The ways in which multiple images are arranged are endless. They are sometimes placed vertically, sometimes horizontally or obliquely, and sometimes in circles, triangles, and other geometrical forms. Their number, too, may vary from two to three, four, or more. They may be stationary or they may change their position more or less rapidly. They also show an infinite variety of colours, including a white even whiter than that of the background.

Illusions of Location

A full stop following a letter on the same horizontal level as the bottom of the letter may appear to change its position in a great variety of curious ways. Its distance from the letter may vary. It may even appear on the other side of the letter. It may also appear above or below the line. Some persons see letters arranged in irregular order. In the case of the word AND, for instance, the D may occupy the place of the N, or the first letter may change places with the last.

All these things are mental illusions. The letters sometimes appear to be farther off than they really are. The small letters, twenty feet distant, may appear to be a mile away. People troubled by illusions of distance sometimes ask if the position of the card has been changed.

Illusions of Nonexistent Objects

When the eye has imperfect sight, the mind not only distorts what the eye sees but imagines that it sees things that do not exist. Among the illusions of this sort are the floating specks which so often appear before the eyes when the sight is imperfect, and even when it is ordinarily very good. These specks are known scientifically as *muscae volitantes*, or 'flying flies', and although they are of no real importance,. being symptoms of nothing except mental strain, they have attracted so much attention and usually cause so much alarm to people that they will be discussed at length in Chapter 19.

Illusions of Complementary Colours

When the sight is imperfect, a person, on looking away from a black, white, or brightly coloured object and closing his eyes, often imagines for a few seconds that he sees the object in a complementary, or approximately complementary, colour. If the object is black upon a white background, a white object upon a black background will be seen. If the object is red it may be seen as blue, and if it is blue it may appear to be red. These illusions which are known as after-images, may also be seen, though less commonly, with the eyes open upon any background at which the subject happens to look, and are often so vivid that they appear to be real.

Illusions of the Colour of the Sun

Persons with normal sight see the sun white, the whitest white there is, but when the sight is imperfect it may appear to be almost any colour in the spectrum—red, green, purple, yellow, etc. In fact, it has even been described by persons with imperfect vision as totally black. The setting sun commonly appears to be red, because of atmospheric conditions, but in many cases these conditions are not enough to change the colour, and while it still appears to be red to persons with imperfect vision, to persons with normal vision it appears to be white. When the redness of a red sun is an illusion and not due to atmospheric conditions, the sun's image on the ground glass of a camera will be white, not red, and the rays focused with a burning glass will also be white. The same is true of a red moon.

Blind Spots After Looking at the Sun

After looking at the sun, most people see black or coloured spots which may last from a few minutes to a year or longer, but are never permanent. These spots are also illusions and are not due, as is commonly supposed, to any organic change in the eye. Even the total blindness which sometimes results temporarily

119

from looking at the sun is only the eye's false impression of a sensory phenomenon.

Illusions of Twinkling Stars

The idea that the stars twinkle has been embodied in song and story, and is generally accepted as part of the natural order of things, but it can be demonstrated that the supposed twinkling is simply an illusion of the mind.

The Cause of the Illusions of Imperfect Sight

All the illusions of imperfect sight are the result of a strain of the mind; when the mind is disturbed for any reason, illusions of all kinds are very likely to occur. Not only is this strain different from the strain that produces the error of refraction, but it can be demonstrated that for every one of these illusions there is a different kind of strain. Alterations of colour do not necessarily affect the size or form of objects or produce any other illusion, and it is possible to see perfectly the colour of a letter, or of a part of a letter, without recognizing the letter. To change black letters into blue, yellow, or another colour, requires a subconscious strain to remember or imagine the colours concerned, while to alter the form requires a subconscious strain to see the form in question. With a little practice anyone can learn to produce illusions of form and colour by straining consciously in the same way that one strains unconsciously, and whenever illusions are produced in this way it will be found that eccentric fixation and an error of refraction have also been produced.

The strain which produces polyopia is different again from the strain which produces illusions of colour, size, and form. After a few attempts most people easily learn to produce polyopia at will. Staring or squinting, if the strain is great enough, will usually make one see double. By looking above a light or a letter and trying to see it as well as when it was directly regarded, one can produce an illusion of several lights or letters, arranged vertically. If the strain is great enough, there may be as many as a dozen of them. By looking to the side of the light or letter, or looking away obliquely at any angle, the images can be made to arrange themselves horizontally, or obliquely at any angle.

To see objects in the wrong location, as when the first letter of a word occupies the place of the last, requires an ingenuity of eccentric fixation and an education of the imagination which is unusual.

The black or coloured spots seen after looking at the sun, and the strange colours which the sun sometimes seems to assume, are also the result of mental strain. When one becomes able to look at the sun without strain (see Chapter 24), these phenomena immediately disappear.

Afterimages have been attributed to fatigue of the retina, which is supposed to have been so overstimulated by a certain colour that it can no longer perceive it and therefore seeks relief in the hue which is complementary to this colour. If it gets tired looking at the black C on a test card, for instance, it is supposed to seek relief by seeing the C white. This explanation of the phenomenon is very ingenious, but scarcely plausible. The eyes cannot see when they are closed, and if they appear to see under these conditions, it is obvious that the subject is suffering from a mental illusion with

121

which the retina has nothing to do. Neither can they see what does not exist, and if, they appear to see a white C on a green wall where there is no such object, it is obvious again that the person is suffering from a mental illusion. The afterimage indicates, in fact, simply a loss of mental control, and occurs when there is an error of refraction, because this condition also is due to a loss of mental control. Anyone can produce an afterimage at will by trying to see the big C all alike—that is, under a strain—but one can look at it indefinitely by central fixation without any such result.

While persons with imperfect sight usually see the stars twinkle, they do not necessarily do so. Therefore it is evident that the strain which causes the twinkling is different from that which causes the error of refraction. If one can look at a star without trying to see it, it does not twinkle; and when the illusion of twinkling has been produced, one can usually stop it by 'swinging' the star. On the other hand, one can make the planets or even the moon twinkle, if one strains sufficiently to see them.

Illusions of Normal Sight

The illusions of normal sight include all the phenomena of central fixation. When the eye with normal sight looks at a letter on a test card it sees best the point fixed, and everything else in the field of vision appears less distinct. As a matter of fact, the whole letter and all the letters may be perfectly black and distinct, and the impression that one letter is blacker than the others, or that one part of a letter is blacker than the rest, is an illusion. The normal eye, however, may shift so rapidly

122

that it appears to see a whole line of small letters all alike simultaneously. As a matter of fact there is, of course, no such picture on the retina. Each letter has been seen separately, and it has been demonstrated in the preceding chapter that if the letters were seen at a distance of fifteen or twenty feet, they could not be recognized unless about four shifts were made on each letter. To produce the impression of a simultaneous picture of fourteen letters, therefore, some sixty or seventy pictures, each with some one point more distinct than the rest, must have been produced upon the retina. The idea that the letters are seen all alike simultaneously is now seen to be an illusion.

Here we have two different kinds of illusions. In the first case the impression made upon the brain is in accordance with the picture on the retina but not in accordance with the fact. In the second the mental impression is in accordance with the fact but not with the pictures upon the retina.

The normal eye usually sees the background of a letter whiter than it really is. In looking at the letters on a test card it sees white streaks at the margins of the letters, and in reading fine print it sees between the lines and the letters, and in the openings of the letters, a white more intense than the reality. Persons who can not read fine print may see this illusion, but less clearly. The more clearly it is seen, the better the vision, and if it can be imagined consciously—it is imagined unconsciously when the sight is normal—the vision improves. If the lines of fine type are covered, the streaks between them disappear. When the letters are seen through a magnifying glass by the eye with normal sight, the illusion is not destroyed but the intensity of the white and black is lessened. With imperfect sight it may be increased to some extent by this means, but will remain less intense than the white and black seen by the normal eye.

The illusions of movement produced by the shifting of the eye and described in detail in the preceding chapter must also be numbered among the illusions of normal sight, and so must the perception of objects in an upright position. This last is the most curious illusion of all. No matter what the position of the head, and regardless of the fact that the image on the retina is inverted, we always see things right side up.

14

Vision Under Adverse Conditions

ACCORDING to the accepted ideas of ocular hygiene, it is important to protect the eyes from a great variety of influences which are often very difficult to avoid, and to which most people resign themselves with the uneasy sense that they are thereby 'ruining their eyesight'. Bright lights, artificial light, dim lights, sudden fluctuations of light, fine print, reading in moving vehicles, reading lying down, and so forth, have long been considered 'bad for the eyes', and libraries of literature have been produced about their supposedly dreadful effects.

These ideas are diametrically opposed to the truth. When the eyes are properly used, vision under adverse conditions not only does not injure them but is an actual benefit, because a greater degree of relaxation is required to see under such conditions than under more favourable ones. It is true that the conditions in question may at first cause discomfort, even to persons with normal vision; but a careful study of the facts has proved that only persons with imperfect sight suffer seriously from them, and that such persons, if they practice central fixation, quickly become accustomed to them and derive great benefit from them.

Although the eyes were made to react to the light, a

very general fear of the effect of this element upon the organs of vision is entertained both by the medical profession and by the laity. When actual disease is present, it is no uncommon thing for people to be kept for weeks, months, and years in dark rooms or with bandages over their eyes.

"A close friend of mine was a branch manager of a nationalised bank for quite some time and whenever I had had an opportunity to meet him I made it a point to enquire of his profession and related activities.

His main complaint always used to be about lack of time for which he held the bank customers responsible. He strongly believed that his customers took away a major part of his working hours leaving very little time to attend to other important activities. He was later on transferred to the administrative side where he had no customers to take away his time. But here too, my friend was in the same predicament—of not getting enough time to do the work allotted to him. His wife, he said, always used to grumble and curse the bank for keeping him so busy throughout the day and making her family life miserable.

Fine Print

The evidence on which this universal fear of light has been based is of the slightest. That brilliant sources of light sometimes produce unpleasant temporary symptoms cannot, of course, be denied; but with regard to definite pathological effects or permanent impairment of vision from exposure to light alone, I have never found, either clinically or experimentally, anything of a positive nature. In my experience strong light has never been permanently injurious.

It is not light but darkness that is dangerous to the eye. Prolonged exclusion from the light always lowers the vision, and may produce serious inflammatory conditions. The universal fear of reading or doing fine work in a dim light is, however, unfounded. As long as the light is strong enough so that one can see without discomfort, this practice is harmless and may be beneficial.

126

Sudden contrasts of light are supposed to be particularly harmful to the eye, but I find no evidence whatever to support this theory. Sudden fluctuations of light undoubtedly cause discomfort to many persons, but, far from being injurious, I have found them in all cases observed to be actually beneficial. Persons with imperfect sight suffer great inconvenience, resulting in lowered vision, from changes in the intensity of the light, but the lowered vision is always temporary, and if the eye is persistently exposed to these conditions the sight is benefitted.

Such practices as reading alternately in a bright and a dim light, or going from a dark room to a well-lighted one and vice versa, are to be recommended. Even such rapid and violent fluctuations of light as those involved in watching a motion picture are, in the long run, beneficial to all eyes. I always advise people with defective vision to go to the movies frequently and practice central fixation. They soon become accustomed to the flickering light, and afterward other light and reflections cause less annoyance.

Reading is supposed to be one of the necessary evils of civilization, but it is believed that by avoiding fine print and taking care to read only under certain favourable conditions, its deleterious influences can be minimized. Extensive investigations as to the effect of various styles of print on the eyesight of schoolchildren have been made, and detailed rules have been laid down as to the size of the print, its shading, the distance of the letters from each other, the spaces between the lines, the length of the lines, and so forth. Children might be bored by books in excessively small print, but I have never seen any reason for supposing that their eyes, or any other eyes, would be harmed by such type. On the contrary, the reading of fine print, when it can be done without discomfort, has invariably proved to be beneficial, and the dimmer the light in which it can be read, and the closer to the eyes it can be held, the greater the benefit. By this means severe pain in the eyes has been relieved in a few minutes or even instantly.

The reason for this is that fine print cannot be read in dim light and close to the eyes unless the eyes are relaxed, whereas large print can be read in a good light and at ordinary reading distance, although the eyes may be under a strain. When fine print can be read under adverse conditions, the reading of ordinary print under ordinary conditions is vastly improved. In myopia it may be a benefit to strain to see fine print, because myopia is always lessened when there is a strain to see near objects, and this has sometimes counteracted the tendency to strain in looking at distant objects, which is always associated with the production of myopia. Even straining to see print so fine that it cannot be read is a benefit to some myopes.

Persons who wish to preserve their eyesight are frequently warned not to read in moving vehicles, but since under modern conditions of life many persons have to spend a large part of their time in moving vehicles, and many of them have no other time to read, it is useless to expect that they will ever discontinue the practice. Fortunately the theory of its injuriousness is not borne out by the facts. When the object regarded is moved more or less rapidly, strain and lowered vision are always produced at first; but this is always temporary, and ultimately the vision is improved by the practice.

There is probably no visual habit against which we have been more persistently warned than that of reading in a recumbent posture. Many plausible reasons have been produced for its supposed injuriousness, but so delightful is the practice that probably few people have ever been deterred from it by fear of the consequences. It is gratifying to be able to state, therefore, that I have found these consequences to be beneficial rather than injurious. As with use of the eyes under other difficult conditions, it is a good thing to be able to read lying down, and the ability to do it improves with practice. In an upright position, with a good light coming over the left shoulder, one can read with the eyes under a considerable degree of strain, but in a recumbent posture, with the light and the angle of the page to the eye unfavourable, one cannot read unless one relaxes. Anyone who can read lying down without discomfort is not likely to have any difficulty in reading under ordinary conditions.

The fact is that vision under difficult conditions is good mental training. The mind may be disturbed at first by the unfavourable environment, but after it has become accustomed to such environments, the mental control and, consequently, the eyesight are improved. The convalescent must not at once try to run a marathon, nor must the person with defective vision attempt, without some preparation, to outstare the sun at noon. But just as the invalid may gradually increase his strength until the marathon has no terrors for him, so may the eye with defective sight be educated until all the rules with which we have so long allowed ourselves to be harassed in the name of 'eye hygiene' may be disregarded, not only with safety but with benefit.

15

Optimums and Pessimums

In nearly all cases of imperfect sight due to errors of refraction there is some object, or objects, which can be regarded with normal vision. Such objects I have called 'optimums'. On the other hand, there are some objects which persons with normal eyes and ordinarily normal sight always see imperfectly, an error of refraction being produced when they are regarded, as demonstrated by the retinoscope. Such objects I have called 'pessimums'. An object becomes an optimum or a pessimum according to the effect it produces upon the mind, and in some cases this effect is easily accounted for.

For many children their mother's face is an optimum, and the face of a stranger a pessimum. A dressmaker was always able to thread a No. 10 needle with a fine thread of silk without glasses, although she had to put on glasses to sew on buttons because she could not see the holes. She was a teacher of dressmaking, and she thought the children stupid because they could not tell the difference between two shades of black. She could match colours without comparing the samples, yet she could not see a black line in a photographic copy of the Bible which was no finer than a thread of silk, and she could not remember a black full stop. An employee in a cooperage, who had been engaged for years in picking out defective barrels as they went rapidly past him on an inclined plane, was able to continue his work after his sight for most other objects had become very defective, while persons with much better sight according to the test card were unable to detect the defective barrels. The familiarity of these various objects made it possible for the subjects to look at them without strain —that is, without trying to see them. Therefore the barrels were optimums to the inspector and the needle's eye and the colours of silk and fabrics were optimums to the dressmaker. Unfamiliar objects, on the contrary, are always pessimums, as pointed out in Chapter 4.

In other cases there is no accounting for the idiosyncrasy of the mind which makes one object a pessimum and another an optimum. It is also impossible to account for the fact that an object may be an optimum for one eye and not for the other, or an optimum at one time and at one distance and not at others. Among these unaccountable optimums one often finds a particular letter on a test card. One patient of mine, for instance, was able to see the letter K on the forty, fifteen and ten lines, but he could see none of the other letters on these lines—although most patients would see some of them, because of the simplicity of their outlines, better than they would such a letter as K.

Pessimums may be as curious and unaccountable as optimums. The letter V is so simple in its outlines that many people can see it when they cannot see others on the same line. Yet some people are unable to distinguish it at any distance, although they can read others in the same word or on the same line of the test card. Some people again will be unable not only to recognize the letter V in a word but also to read any word that contains it, the pessimum lowering their sight both for itself and for other objects.

Some letters, or objects, become pessimums only in particular situations. A letter, for instance, may be a pessimum when located at the end or the beginning of a line or a sentence, and not in other places. When the attention of the patient is called to the fact that a letter seen in one location ought logically to be seen just as well in others, the letter often ceases to be a pessimum in any situation.

A pessimum, like an optimum, may be lost and later become manifest. It may vary according to the light and distance. An object which is a pessimum in a moderate light may not be so when the light is increased or diminished. A pessimum at twenty feet may not be one not' at two feet or thirty feet, and an object which is a pessimum when directly regarded may be seen with normal vision in the eccentric field.

For most people the test card is a pessimum. If you can see it with normal vision, you can see almost anything else in the world. Patients who cannot see the letters on the test card can often see other objects of the same size and at the same distance with normal sight. When letters which are seen imperfectly, or even letters which cannot be seen at all, or which a person is not conscious of seeing, are regarded, the error of refraction is increased. A person may look at a blank white card without any error of refraction, but if he looks at the lower part of a test card, which appears to him to be just as the blank card, an error of refraction can always be demonstrated, and if the visible letters of the card are covered, the result is the same. The pessimum may, in short, be letters or objects which the

132

person is not conscious of seeing. This phenomenon is very common.

When the card is seen in the eccentric field, it may have the effect of lowering the vision for the point directly regarded. For instance, a person may regard an area of green wallpaper at the distance and see the colour as well as at the near-point; but if a test card on which the letters are seen either imperfectly or not at all is placed in the neighbourhood of the area being regarded, the retinoscope may indicate an error of refraction. When the vision improves, the number of letters on the card which are pessimums diminishes and the number of optimums increases, until the whole card becomes an optimum.

A pessimum, like an optimum, is a manifestation of the mind. It is something associated with a strain to see, just as an optimum is something which has no such association. It is not caused by the error of refraction, but always produces an error of refraction, and when the strain has been relieved it ceases to be a pessimum and becomes an optimum.

16

Presbyopia: Its Cause and Treatment

AMONG people living under civilized conditions the accommodative power of the eye gradually declines, in most cases, until at the age of sixty or seventy it appears to have been entirely lost, a person being absolutely dependent upon his glasses for vision at the near-point. As to whether the same thing happens among primitive people or people living under primitive conditions, very little information is available. Some ophthalmologists think that the power of accommodation does not diminish, if at all, more rapidly among people who use their eyes a great deal at the near-point than among agriculturists, sailors, and people who use them mainly for distant vision; others say the opposite.

It is a fact, however, that people who cannot read, no matter what their age, will manifest a failure of near vision if asked to look at printed characters, although their sight for familiar objects at the near-point may be perfect. That such persons, at the age of forty-five or fifty, cannot differentiate between printed characters is no warrant, therefore, for the conclusion that their accommodative powers are declining. A young illiterate would do no better, and a young student who can read Roman characters at the near-point without difficulty always develops symptoms or imperfect sight when he attempts to read old English, Greek, or Chinese characters for the first time.

When the accommodative power has declined to the point at which reading and writing become difficult, the person is said to have presbyopia, or, more popularly, 'old sight'. The condition is generally accepted, by both the popular and the scientific mind, as one of the unavoidable inconveniences of old age.

The decline of accommodative power with advancing years is commonly attributed to the hardening of the lens, an influence which is believed to be augmented in later years by a flattening of this body and a lowering of its refractive status, together with weakness or atrophy of the ciliary muscle. So regular is the decline, in most cases, that tables have been compiled showing the near-point to be expected at various ages. From these it is said one might almost fit glasses without testing the vision of a person, or, conversely, one might judge a man's age within a year or two from his glasses.

According to the depressing figures of one of these tables, one must expect at thirty to have lost no less than half of one's original accommodative power, while at forty two-thirds of it is gone, and at sixty it is practically non-existent.

There are many people, however, who do not fit this schedule. Many persons at forty can read fine print at four inches, although they ought, according, to the table, to have lost that power shortly after becoming twenty years old. Worse still, there are people who refuse to become presbyopic at all. Oliver Wendell Holmes mentions one of these cases in *The Autocrat of the Breakfast Table*.

135

'There is now living in New York State', he said, an old gentleman who, perceiving his sight to fail, immediately took to exercising it on the finest print, and in this way fairly bullied Nature out of her foolish habit of taking liberties at five-and-forty, or thereabout. And now this old gentleman performs the most extraordinary feats with his pen, showing that his eyes must be a pair of microscopes. I should be afraid to say how much he writes in the compass of a half-dime—whether the Psalms or the Gospels, or the Psalms and the Gospels, I won't be positive.

There are also people who regain their near vision after having lost it for ten, fifteen, or more years, and there are people who, while presbyopic for some objects, have perfect sight for others. Many dressmakers, for instance, can thread a needle with the naked eye, and with the retinoscope it can be demonstrated that they accurately focus their eyes upon such objects; and yet they cannot read or write without glasses.

So far as I am aware, no one but myself has ever observed the last-mentioned class of cases, but the others are known to every ophthalmologist of any experience. One hears of them at the meetings of ophthalmological societies, they are even reported in the medical journals; but such is the force of authority that when it comes to writing books they are either ignored or explained away, and most of the new treatises that come from the press repeat the old superstition that presbyopia is 'a normal result of growing old.' The dead hand of German science still oppresses our intellects and prevents us from crediting the plainest evidence of our senses. German ophthalmology is still sacred, and no facts are allowed to cast discredit upon it.

Fortunately for those who feel called upon to defend the old theories, myopia postpones are advent of presbyopia, and a decrease in the size of the pupil, which often takes place in old age, has some effect in facilitating vision at the near-point. Reported cases of persons reading without glasses when over fifty or fifty-five years of age, therefore, can be easily disposed of by assuming that the subject must be myopic, or that their pupils are unusually small. If the case comes under actual observation, the matter may not be so simple, because it may be found that the person, far from being myopic, is hypermetropic or emmetropic, and that the pupil is of normal size. There is nothing to do with these cases but to ignore them.

Abnormal changes in the form of the lens have also been held responsible for the retention of near vision beyond the prescribed age, or for its restoration after it has been lost, the swelling of the lens in incipient cataract affording a very convenient and plausible explanation for the latter class of cases. In cases of premature presbyopia, 'accelerated sclerosis' of the lens and weakness of the ciliary muscle have been assumed; and if cases like that of the dressmakers who can thread their needles when they can no longer read the newspapers had been observed, no doubt some explanation consistent with the German view-point would have been found for them.

The truth about presbyopia is that it is not 'a normal result of growing old', because it can be both prevented and eliminated. It is caused not by a hardening of the lens but by a strain to see at the near-point. It has no necessary connection with age, since it occurs in some cases as early as the age of ten, while in others it never occurs at all, although the person may live far into the

137

so-called presbyopic age. It is true that the lens does harden with advancing years, just as the bones harden and the structure of the skin changes, but since the lens is not a factor in accommodation, this fact is immaterial. Also, while in some cases the lens may become flatter or lose some of its refractive power with advancing years, it has been observed to remain perfectly clear and unchanged in shape up to the age of ninety. Since the ciliary muscle is not a factor in accommodation either, its weakness or atrophy can contribute nothing to the decline of accommodative power.

Presbyopia is, in fact, simply a form of hypermetropia in which the vision for the near-point is chiefly affected, although the vision for the distance, contrary to what is generally believed, is always lowered too. The difference between the two conditions is not always clear. A person with hypermetropia may or may not read fine print, and a person at the presbyopic age may read it without apparent inconvenience and yet have imperfect sight for the distance. In both conditions the sight at both points is lowered, although the person may be aware of it.

It has been shown that when the eyes strain to see at the near-point, the focus is always pushed farther away than it was before, in one or all meridians. By means of simultaneous retinoscopy it can be demonstrated that when a person with presbyopia tries to read fine print and fails, the focus is always pushed farther away than it was before the attempt was made, indicating that the failure was caused by strain. Even the thought of making such an effort will produce strain, so that the refraction may be changed and pain, discomfort and fatigue produced, before the fine print is regarded.

138

Furthermore, when a person with presbyopia rests his eyes by closing them or palming, he always becomes able, for a few moments at least, to read fine print at six inches, again indicating that his previous failure was due not to any fault of the eyes but to a strain to see. When the strain is permanently relieved, the presbyopia is permanently eliminated; this has happened not in a few cases but in many, and at all ages up to sixty, seventy, and eighty.

The first patient that I cured of presbyopia was myself. Having demonstrated by means of experiments on the eyes of animals that the lens is not a factor in accommodation, I knew that presbyopia must be remediable. But I realized that I could not look for any very general acceptance of the revolutionary conclusions I had reached as long as I wore glasses myself for a condition supposed to be due to the loss of the accommodative power of the lens.

I was then suffering from the maximum degree of presbyopia. I had no accommodative power whatever and had to have quite an outfit of glasses, because with a glass which enabled me to read fine print at thirteen inches, for instance, I could not read it either at twelve inches or at fourteen. The retinoscope showed that when I tried to see anything at the near-point without glasses my eyes were focused for the distance, and when I tried to see anything at the distance they were focused for the near-point.

My problem, then, was to find some way of reversing this condition and inducing my eyes to focus for the point I wished to see at the moment that I wished to see it. I consulted various eye specialists, but my language was to them like that of St. Paul to the Greeks, foolishness.

'Your lens is as hard as a stone,' they said. 'No one can do anything for you.'

Then I went to a nerve specialist. He used the retinoscope on me and confirmed my own observations as to the peculiar contrariness of my accommodation, but he had no idea what I could do about it. He would consult some of his colleagues, he said, and asked me to come back in a month, which I did. Then he told me he had come to the conclusion that there was only one man who could cure me, and that was Dr William H. Bates of New York.

'Why do you say that?' I asked.

'Because you are the only man who seems to know anything about it,' he answered.

Thus thrown upon my own resources, I was fortunate enough to find a nonmedical gentleman who was willing to do what he could to assist me. He kindly used the retinoscope through many long and tedious hours, while I studied my own case and tried to find some way of accommodating when I wanted to read instead of when I wanted to see something at the distance.

One day, while looking at a picture of the Rock of Gibraltar which hung on the wall, I noted some black spots on its face. I imagined that these spots were the openings of caves and that there were people in these caves moving about. When I did this my eyes were focused for the reading distance. Then I looked at the same picture at the reading distance, still imagining that the spots were caves with people in them. The retinoscope showed that I had accommodated, and I was able to read the lettering beside the picture, I had, in fact, been temporarily helped by the use of my imagination.

Later I found that when I imagined the letters black I was able to see them black, and when I saw them black I was able to distinguish their form. My progress after this was not what could be called rapid. It was six months before I could read the newspapers with any kind of comfort, and a year before I obtained my present accommodative range of fourteen inches from four inches to eighteen. But the experience was extremely valuable, for I had in pronounced form every symptom subsequently observed in other presbyopic patients.

Fortunately for my patients, it has seldom taken me as long to relieve other people as it did to relieve myself. In some cases a complete and permanent correction was effected in a few minutes. One patient who had worn glasses for presbyopia for about twenty years was improved in less than fifteen minutes by the use of his imagination.

In this latter case, when the patient was asked to read diamond type he said he could not do so because the letters were grey and looked all alike. I reminded him that the type was printer's ink and that there was nothing blacker than that. I asked him if he had ever seen printer's ink. He replied that he had. Did he remember how black it was? Yes. Did he believe that these letters were as black as the ink he remembered? He did, and then he read the letters—and because the improvement in his vision was permanent, he said that I hypnotized him.

In another case, a presbyope of ten years' standing was relieved just as quickly by the same method. When reminded that the letters which he could not read were black, he replied that he knew they were black but that they looked grey.

141

'If you know they are black and yet you see them grey,' I said, 'you must imagine them grey. Suppose you imagine that they are black. Can you do that?'

'Yes,' he said 'I can imagine that they are black.' Then he proceeded to read them.

These extremely quick restorations are rare. In nine cases out of ten, progress has been much slower and it has been necessary to resort to all the methods of obtaining relaxation found useful in the treatment of other errors of refraction. In the more difficult cases of presbyopia people often suffer from the same illusions of colour, size, form and number when they try to read fine print as do people with hypermetropia, astigmatism, and myopia when they try to read the letters on a test card at the distance. They are unable to remember or imagine, when trying to see at the near-point, even such a simple thing as a small black spot, but they can remember it perfectly when they do not try to see. Their sight for the distance is often very imperfect and always below normal, although they may have thought it perfect; and just as in the case of other errors of refraction, improvement of the distant vision improves the vision at the near-point. Regardless, however, of the difficulty of the case and the age of the person, some improvement has always been obtained, and if the treatment was continued long enough completely normal sight was attained.

The idea that presbyopia is a normal result of growing old is responsible for much defective eyesight. When people who have reached the presbyopic age experience difficulty in reading, they are very likely to resort at once to glasses, either with or without professional advice. In some cases such persons may be actually presbyopic; in others the difficulty may be something temporary, which they would have thought little about if they had been younger, and which would have passed away if Nature had been left to herself. But once the glasses are adopted, in the great majority of cases, they produce the condition they were designed to relieve or, if it already existed, they make it worse, sometimes very rapidly, as every ophthalmologist knows.

In a few weeks, sometimes, the person finds as noted in Chapter 5, that the large print which he could read without difficulty before he got his glasses can no longer be read without their aid. In from five to ten years the accommodative power of the eye is usually gone, and if from this point the person does not go on to cataract, glaucoma, or inflammation of the retina, he may consider himself fortunate.

Only occasionally do the eyes refuse to submit to the artificial conditions imposed upon them, but in such cases they may keep up an astonishing struggle against them for long periods. A woman of seventy who had worn glasses for twenty years was still able to read diamond type and had good vision for the distance without them. She said the glasses tired her eyes and blurred her vision, but that she had persisted in wearing them, in spite of a continual temptation to throw them off, because she had been told that it was necessary for her to do so.

If persons who find themselves getting presbyopic, or who have arrived at the presbyopic age, would, instead of resorting to glasses, follow the example of the gentleman mentioned by Dr Holmes and make a practice of reading the finest print they can find, the idea that the decline of accommodative power is 'a normal result of growing old' would soon die a natural death.

17

Squint and Amblyopia: Their Cause

SINCE we have two eyes, it is obvious that in the act of sight two pictures must be formed. In order that these two pictures shall be fused into one by the mind, it is necessary that there shall be perfect harmony of action between the two organs of vision. In looking at a distant object the two visual axes must be parallel, and in looking at an object at a distance less than infinity, which for practical purposes is less than twenty feet, they must converge to exactly the same degree.

The absence of this harmony of action is known as strabismus, or squint, and is one of the most distressing of eye defects, not only because of the lowering of vision involved but because the lack of symmetry in the most expressive feature of the face which results from it has a most unpleasant effect upon personal appearance. The condition is one which has long baffled ophthalmological science. While the theories about its cause that are advanced in the textbooks seem to fit some cases, they leave others unexplained, and all methods of treatment are admitted to be very uncertain in their results.

The idea that a lack of harmony in the movements of the eye is due to a corresponding lack of harmony in the strength of the muscles that turn them in their sockets seemed such a natural one that this theory was almost universally accepted at one time. Operations based upon it once had a great vogue, but today they are advised, by most authorities, only as a last resort. It is true that many persons have been benefitted by them, but at best the correction of the squint is only approximate, and in many cases the condition has been made worse, while a restoration of binocular vision—the power of fusing the two visual images into one—is scarcely even hoped for.

Actually, the muscle theory fitted the facts so badly that when it was suggested that squint was a condition growing out of refractive errors—hypermetropia being held responsible for the production of convergent squint and myopia for divergent squint—it was universally accepted. This theory, too, proved unsatisfactory, and now medical opinion is divided between various theories. One attributes the condition, in the great majority of cases, to a defect not of the muscles but of the nerve supply, and it has had many supporters. Another lays stress on the lack of a so-called fusion faculty, and recommends the use of prisms or other measures to develop it. A third states that the anomaly results from a wrong shape of the orbit, and, as it is impossible to alter this condition, advocates operations for the purpose of neutralizing its influence.

In order to make any of these theories appear consistent, it is necessary to explain away a great many troublesome facts. The uncertain result of operations upon the eye muscles is sufficient to cast suspicion on the theory that the condition is due to any abnormality of the muscles, and many cases of marked paralysis of one or more muscles have been observed in which there was no squint. Relief of paralysis, moreover, may not relieve the squint, nor the relief of the squint the paralysis. One outstanding ophthalmologist found so many cases which were not benefitted by training designed to improve the fusion faculty that he recommended operations on the muscles in such cases; another, noting that the majority of hypermetropes did not squint, was obliged to assume that hypermetropia did not cause this condition without the aid of co-operating circumstances.

That the state of the vision is not an important factor in the production of squint is attested by a multitude of facts. It is true that squint is usually associated with errors of refraction, but some people squint with a very slight error of refraction. It is also true that many persons with convergent squint have hypermetropia, while many others have not. Some persons with convergent squint have myopia. A person may also have convergent squint with one eye normal and one hypermetropic myopic, or with one eye blind.

Usually the vision of the eye that turns in is less than that of the eye which is straight, yet there are cases in which the eye with the poorer vision is straight and the eye with the better vision turned in. With two blind eyes, both eyes may be straight, or one may turn in. With one good eye and one blind eye, both eyes may be straight. The blinder the eye, as a rule, the more marked the squint; but exceptions are frequent, and in rare cases an eye with nearly normal vision may turn in persistently.

A squint may also disappear and return again, while convergent squint will change into divergent squint and back again. With the same error of refraction, one person will have squint and another not. A third will squint with a different eye. A fourth will squint first with one eye and then with the other. In a fifth the amount of the squint will vary. One will get well without glasses or other treatment, and another with these aids. These cures may be temporary or permanent, and the relapses may occur either with or without glasses.

However slight the error of refraction, the vision of many squinting eyes is inferior to that of the straight eye, and usually no apparent or sufficient cause for this condition can be found in the constitution of the eye. There is a difference of opinion as to whether this curious defect of vision is the result of the squint or the squint the result of it; but the predominating opinion that it is at least aggravated by the squint has been crystallized in the name given to the condition, *amblyopia ex anopsia*, literally 'dimsightedness from disuse'—for the mind is believed to suppress the image of the deviating eye in order to avoid the annoyance of double vision. There are, however, many squinting eyes without amblyopia, and such a condition has been found in eyes that have never squinted.

The literature of the subject is full of the impossibility of curing amblyopia, and in popular writings persons having the care of children are urged to have cases of squint treated early, so that the vision of the squinting eye may not be lost. According to one eminent ophthalmologist, not much improvement can ordinarily be obtained in amblyopic eyes after the age of six, while another says, 'The function of the retina never again becomes perfectly normal, even if the cause of the visual disturbance is done away with.' Yet it is well known that if the sight of the good eye is lost at any period of life, the vision of the amblyopic eye will often become normal. Furthermore, an eye may be amblyopic at one time and not at another. When the good eye is covered, a squinting eye may be so amblyopic that it can scarcely distinguish daylight from darkness, but when both eyes are open, the vision of the squinting eye may be found to be as good as that of the straight eye, if not better. In many cases, too, the amblyopia will change from one eye to the other.

Double vision occurs very seldom in squint, and when it does, it often assumes very curious forms. When the eyes turn in, the image seen by the right eye should, according to all the laws of optics, be to the right, and the image seen by the left eye to the left. When the eyes turn out, the opposite should be the case. But often the position of the images is reversed, the image of the right eye in convergent squint being seen to the left and that of the left eye to the right, while in divergent squint the opposite is the case. This condition is known as 'paradoxical diplopia'. Furthermore, persons with almost normal vision and both eyes perfectly straight may have both kinds of double vision.

All the theories heretofore suggested fail to explain the foregoing facts, but it is true that in all cases of squint a strain can be demonstrated, and that the relief of the strain is in all cases followed by the disappearance of the squint, as well as of the amblyopia and the error of refraction. It is also true that all persons with normal eyes can produce squint by strain to see. It is not a difficult thing to do, and many children derive amusement from the practice, while it gives their elders unnecessary concern, for fear that the temporary squint may become permanent.

To produce convergent squint is comparatively easy. Children usually do it by straining to see the end of the nose. The production of divergent squint is more difficult, but with practice persons with normal eyes become able to turn out either eye, or both, at will. They also become able to turn either eye upward and inward, or upward and outward, at any desired angle. Any kind of squint can, in fact be produced at will by the appropriate kind of strain. There is usually a lowering of the vision when voluntary squint is produced, and accepted methods of measuring the strength of the muscles seem to show deficiencies corresponding to the nature of the squint.

18

Squint and Amblyopia: Their Treatment

THE evidence is conclusive that squint and amblyopia, like errors of refraction, are purely functional troubles, and since they are always relieved by the relief of the strain with which they are associated, it follows that any of the methods which promote relaxation and central fixation may be employed for their elimination. As in the case of errors of refraction, the squint disappears and the amblyopia is corrected just as soon as a person gains enough mental control to remember a perfectly black full stop. In this way both conditions may be temporarily relieved in a few seconds, their permanent eradication being a mere matter of making this temporary state permanent

One of the best ways of gaining mental control in cases of squint is to learn how to increase the squint, or produce other kinds of squint, voluntarily. A case in point is that of a woman who had divergent vertical squint in both eyes. When the left eye was straight the right eye turned out and up, and when the right eye was straight the left eye turned down and out. Both eyes were amblyopic and there was double vision, with the images sometimes on the same side and sometimes on opposite sides. She suffered from headaches and obtained no relief from glasses or other methods of treatment, so she made up her mind to an operation and consulted a surgeon with the idea of having one performed. The surgeon, puzzled to find so many muscles apparently at fault, asked my opinion as to which of them should be operated upon.

I showed the woman how to make her squint worse, and recommended that the surgeon treat her by eye education without an operation. He did so, and in less than a month the woman had learned to turn both eyes involuntarily. At first she did this by looking at a pencil held over the bridge of her nose, but later she became able to do it without the pencil, and ultimately she learned to produce every kind of squint at will. The treatment was not pleasant for her because the production of new kinds of squint, or the making worse of the existing condition, gave her pain, but it effected a complete and permanent relief both of the squint and of the amblyopia. The same method has proved successful with other people.

Some people do not know whether they are looking straight at an object or not. They may be helped by another person's watching the deviating eye and directing them to look more nearly in the proper direction. When the deviating eye looks directly at an object, the strain to see is less and the vision is consequently improved. Covering the good eye with an opaque screen or with ground glass encourages a more proper use of the squinting eye, especially if the vision of that eye is imperfect.

In the case of children six years old or younger, squint can usually be remedied by the use of atropine, a one per cent solution being instilled into one or both eyes twice a day, for many months, a year, or longer. Atropine makes it more difficult for the child to see and makes the sunlight disagreeable. In order to overcome this handicap the child has to relax, and the relaxation cures the squint.

The improvement resulting from eye education in cases of squint and amblyopia is sometimes so rapid as to be almost incredible. The following are a few of the many examples that might be quoted.

A girl of eleven had convergent vertical squint of the left eye. The vision of this eye at the distance was 3/200, while at the near-point it was so imperfect that she was unable to read. The vision of the right eye was normal for both the near-point and the distance. She was wearing glasses when she came to my office, but had obtained no benefit from them. When she looked three feet away from the big C with the left eye she saw it better than when she looked directly at it, but when I asked her to count my fingers held three feet away from the card, they so attracted her attention that she was able to see the large letter worse. The fact was impressed upon her that when she looked away from the card she could see it better or worse at will, and she was asked to note that when she saw it worse her vision improved and when she saw it better her vision declined. After shifting from the card to a point three feet away from it and seeing the former worse a few times, her vision improved to 10/200.

Her ability to shift and see worse improved by practice so rapidly that in less than ten days her vision was normal in both eyes, and in less than two weeks it had improved to 20/10, while diamond type was read with each eye at from three inches to twenty inches. In less than three weeks her vision for the distance was 20/5, by artificial light, and she read photographic type reductions at two inches, the tests being made with both eyes together and with each eye separately. She also read strange test cards as readily as the familiar ones. She was advised to continue the treatment at home to prevent a relapse, and at the end of three years none had occurred. During the treatment at the office and practice at home the good eye was covered with an opaque screen, but this was not worn at other times.

A similar case was that of a girl of fourteen who had squinted from childhood. The internal rectus muscle of the right eye had been cut when she was two years old, but it still pulled the eye inward. The girl objected to wearing a ground glass over her good eye because her friends teased her about it, and she thought it made her more conspicuous than the squint. One day she lost her glasses in the snow, but her father immediately provided another pair. Then she announced that she was ill and couldn't go to school. I told the father that his daughter was hysterical and simply imagined she was ill in order to avoid treatment. He insisted that she continue, and as she did not consider herself well enough to come to see me, I called upon her.

With the assistance of her father she was made to understand that she would have to continue the treatment, and she at once went to work with such energy and intelligence that in half an hour the vision of the squinting and amblyopic eye had improved from 3/200 to 20/30. She also became able to read fine print at twelve inches. She went back to school wearing the ground glass over the good eye, but whenever she wanted to see she looked over the top of it. Her father followed her to school and insisted that she use the poorer eye instead of the better one. She became convinced that the simplest way out of her troubles would be to follow my instructions, and in less than a

153

week the squint was corrected and she had normal vision in both eyes. At the beginning of the treatment she could not count her fingers at three feet with the poorer eye, and in three weeks, including all the time that she wasted, she had no more trouble at all. When she was told that this was so, her main concern seemed to be to know whether she would have to wear the ground glass any more. She was assured that she would not have to unless there was a relapse, but there never was any relapse.

In a third case a girl of eight had amblyopia and squint since childhood. The vision of the right eye was 10/40, that of the left eye 20/30. Glasses did not improve either eye. The child was seated twenty feet from a test card and the right, or poorer, eye was covered with an opaque screen. She was directed to look with her better eye at the large letter on the card and to note its clearness. Next she was told to look at a point three feet to one side of the card, and her attention was called to the fact that she did not see the large letter so well then. The point of fixation was brought closer and closer to the letter, until she appreciated the fact that her vision was lowered when she looked only a few inches to one side of it. When she looked at a small letter she readily recognized that an eccentric fixation of less than an inch lowered her vision.

After she had learned to increase the amblyopia of the better eye, this eye was covered while she was taught how to lower the vision of the other, or poorer, eye by increasing its eccentric fixation. This was accomplished in a few minutes. She was told that the cause of her defective sight was her habit of looking at objects with a part of the retina to one side of the true centre of sight. She was advised to see by looking

154

straight at the test card. In less than half an hour the vision of the left eye became normal, while the right improved from 10/40 to 10/10. Her vision was normal in two weeks.

19

Floating Specks: Their Cause and Treatment

A VERY common phenomenon of imperfect sight is that
one, already mentioned, which is known as *muscae volitantes*, or flying flies. These floating specks are usually
dark or black, but sometimes appear as white bubbles,
and in rare cases many assume all the colours of
the rainbow. They move somewhat rapidly, usually in curving lines, before the eyes, and always
appear to be just beyond the point of fixation. If one
tries to look at them directly, they seem to move a little
farther away. Hence their name.

The literature on the subject is full of speculations
as to the origin of these appearances. Some have
attributed them to the presence of floating specks—
dead cells or the debris of cells—in the vitreous humour
the transparent substance that fills four-fifths of the
eyeball behind the crystalline lens. Similar specks on
the surface of the cornea have also been held responsible for them. It has even been surmised that they
might be caused by the passage of tears over the
cornea.

They are so common in myopia that they have been
supposed to be one of the symptoms of this condition,
although they occur also with other errors of refraction
as well as in eyes otherwise normal. They have been

attributed to disturbances of the circulation, the digestion, and the kidneys. and because so many insane people have them, they have been thought to be an evidence of incipient insanity. The patent-medicine business has thrived upon them, and it would be difficult to estimate the amount of mental torture they have caused, as the following cases illustrate.

A clergyman who was much annoyed by the continual appearance of floating specks before his eyes was told by his eye specialist that they were a symptom of kidney disease, and that in many cases of kidney trouble disease of the retina might be an early symptom. So at regular intervals he went to the specialist to have his eyes examined, and when at length the doctor died he looked around immediately for someone else to make the periodical examination. His family physician directed him to me.

I was by no means as well known as his previous ophthalmological adviser, but it happened that I had taught the family physician how to use the ophthalmoscope after others had failed to do so. He thought, therefore, that I must know a lot about the use of the instrument, and what the clergyman particularly wanted was someone capable of making a thorough examination of the interior of his eyes and detecting at once any signs of kidney disease that might make their appearance. So he came to me, and I made a very careful examination of his eyes. He went away happy because I could find nothing wrong but he came back periodically just for a check-up.

Once when I was out of town, however, he got a cinder in his eye and went to another oculist to get it out. When I came back late at night I found him sitting on my doorstep, on the chance that I might return.

His story was a pitiful one. The new doctor had examined his eyes with the ophthalmoscope and had suggested the possibility of glaucoma, describing the disease as a very treacherous one which might make him go blind suddenly and which would be agonizingly painful. He emphasized what the patient had previously been told about the danger of kidney disease, suggested that the liver and heart might also be involved, and advised him to have all of these organs carefully examined.

I made another examination of the clergyman's eyes in general and their tension in particular; I had him feel his eyeballs and compare them with my own, so that he might see for himself that they were not becoming hard as a stone; and finally I succeeded in reassuring him.

In another case that came to my attention, a man returning from Europe was looking at some white clouds one day when floating specks appeared before his eyes. He consulted the ship's doctor, who told him that the symptom was very serious and might be the forerunner of blindness. It might also indicate incipient insanity, as well as other nervous or organic diseases. He was advised to consult his family physician and an eye specialist as soon as he landed, which he did.

This was twenty-five years ago, but I shall never forget the terrible state of nervousness and terror into which the man had worked himself by the time he came to me. It was even worse than that of the clergyman, who was always ready to admit that his fears were unreasonable. I examined this man's eyes very carefully and found them absolutely normal. The vision was perfect for both the near-point and the distance. The colour perception, the fields, and the tension were normal, and under a strong magnifying glass I could find no opacities in the vitreous. In short, there were absolutely no symptoms of any disease.

I told the man there was nothing wrong with his eyes, and I also showed him an advertisement for a quack medicine in a newspaper, which gave a great deal of space to describing the dreadful things likely to follow the appearance of floating specks before the eyes unless one began betimes to take the medicine in question at one dollar a bottle. I pointed out that the advertisement, which was appearing in all the big newspapers of the city every day, and probably in other cities, must have cost a lot of money and must therefore be bringing in a lot of money. Evidently there must be a great many people suffering from this symptom, and if it were as serious as was generally believed, there would be a great many more blind and insane people in the community than there actually were.

My patient went away somewhat comforted, but at eleven o'clock—his first visit had been at nine—he was back again. He still saw the floating specks, and was still worried about them. I examined his eyes again as carefully as before, and again was able to assure him that there was nothing wrong with them. In the afternoon I was not in my office, but I was told that he was there at three o'clock and at five. At seven he came again, bringing with him his family physician, an old friend of mine. I said to the latter:

Please make this man stay at home. I have to charge him for his visits, because he is taking up so much of my time, but it is a shame to take his money when there is nothing wrong with him.'

What my friend said to him I don't know, but he did not come back again.

159

I did not know as much about *muscae volitantes* then as I know now, or I might have saved both of the men just described a great deal of uneasiness. I could tell them that their eyes were normal, but I did not know how to relieve them of the symptoms, which is simply an illusion resulting from mental strain. The specks are associated to a considerable extent with markedly imperfect eyesight, because persons whose eyesight is imperfect always strain to see; but persons whose eyesight is ordinarily normal may see them at times, because no eye has normal sight all the time. Most people can see *muscae volitantes* when they look at the sun or any uniformly bright surface, such as a sheet of white paper upon which the sun is shining. This is because most people strain when they look at surfaces of this kind.

The specks are never seen, in other words, except when the eyes and mind are under a strain, and they always disappear when the strain is relieved. If one can remember a small letter on a test card by central fixation, the specks will immediately disappear or cease to move, but if one tries to remember two or more letters equally well at one time, they will reappear and move.

Usually the strain that causes *muscae volitantes* is very easily relieved. A school teacher who had been annoyed by these appearances for years once came to me because the condition had recently grown much worse. In half an hour I was able to improve her sight, which had been slightly myopic, to normal, whereupon the specks disappeared. Next day they came back, but another visit to the office brought relief. After that the teacher was able to carry out the treatment at home, and had no more trouble.

A physician who suffered constantly from headaches and *muscae volitantes* was able to read only 20/70 when he looked at the test card, while the retinoscope showed mixed astigmatism and he saw the specks. When he looked at a blank wall, or a blank white card, the retinoscope still showed mixed astigmatism and he still saw the specks. But when he remembered a black spot as well as he could see it, when looking at these surfaces, there were no specks, and the retinoscope indicated no error of refraction. In a few days he obtained complete relief from the astigmatism, the *muscae volitantes*, and the headaches, as well as from chronic conjuctivitis (inflammation of the conjuctiva of the eye). His eyes, which had been partly closed, opened wide, and the sclera became white and clear. He became able to read in trains with no inconvenience, and—what impressed him more than anything else—he also became able to sit up all night with patients without having any trouble with his eyes the next day.

20

Home Treatment

IT is not always possible for people to go to a competent physician for relief. As the method of treating eye defects presented in this book is comparatively new, it may be impossible to find a physician in the neighbourhood who understands it, and a person may not be able to afford the expense of a long journey or take the time for treatment away from home. To such persons I wish to say that it is possible for a large number of people to correct defective eyesight without the aid either of a physician or of anyone else. They can improve their own sight, and for this purpose it is not even necessary that they should understand all that has been written in this book, or in any other book. All that is necessary is to follow a few simple directions.

Place a test card on the wall at a distance of ten, fourteen, or twenty feet, and devote half a minute a day, or longer, to reading the smallest letters you can see, with each eye separately, covering the other with the palm of the hand in such a way as to avoid touching the eyeball. Keep a record of the progress made with the dates. The simplest way to do this is by the method used by oculists, who record the vision in the form of a fraction, with the distance at which the letter is read as

162

the numerator and the distance at which it ought to be read as the denominator.

The figures above or to one side of the lines of letters on the test card indicate the distance at which these letters should be read by persons with normal eyesight. Thus a vision of 10/200 would mean that the big C, which on a standard-size chart ought to be read at two hundred feet, cannot be seen at a greater distance than ten feet. A vision of 20/10 would mean that the ten line, which the normal eye is not ordinarily expected to read at a greater distance than ten feet, is seen at twice that distance. This is a standard commonly attained by persons who have practised my methods.

Another and an even better way to test the sight is to compare the blackness of the letter at the near-point and at the distance, in a dim light and in a good one. With perfect sight, as I have explained, black is not altered by illumination or distance. It appears just as black at the distance as at the near-point, and just as black in a dim light as in a good one. If it does not appear equally black to you under all these conditions, therefore, you may know that your sight is imperfect.

Children under twelve years of age who have not worn glasses can usually correct defective eyesight by the above method in three months, six months, or a year. Adults who have never worn glasses are benefitted in a very short time—a week or two—and if the trouble is not very bad, it may be removed in three to six months. Children or adults who have worn glasses, however, are more difficult to relieve, and they usually have to practice the methods of gaining relaxation described in other chapters of this book. They also have to devote considerable time to the treatment.

It is absolutely necessary that the glasses be discarded. No halfway measures can be tolerated, if complete relief is desired. Do not attempt to wear weaker glasses, and do not wear glasses for emergencies. Persons who are unable to do without glasses for all purposes are not likely to be able to cure themselves.

Children and adults who have worn glasses will have to devote an hour or longer every day to practise with the test card, and additional time to practise on other objects. It is well to have two test cards, one to be used at the near-point, where it can be seen best, and the other at ten or twenty feet. It will be found very helpful to shift from the near card to the distant one, as the unconscious memory of the letters seen at the near-point helps to bring out those seen at the distance.

If you can secure the aid of some person with normal sight, it will be great advantage. In fact, persons whose cases are obstinate will find it very difficult, if not impossible, to cure themselves without the aid of a teacher. The teacher, if he is to be of help, must himself be able to derive benefit from the various methods recommended. If his vision is 10/10, he must be able to improve it to 20/10, or more. If he can read fine print at twelve inches, he must become able to read it at six, or at three inches. He must also have sufficient control over his visual memory to relieve and prevent pain. A person who has defective sight, either for the distance or for the near-point, will be unable to be of any material assistance in obstinate cases, and no one can be of any assistance in the application of any method which he himself has not used successfully.

Parents who wish to preserve and improve the eyesight of their children should encourage them to read the test card every day. There should be a test card in every family, in fact, for when properly used it always prevents myopia and other errors of refraction, always improves the vision, even when this is already normal, and always benefits functional nervous troubles. Parents should improve their own eyesight to normal, so that their children may not imitate wrong methods of using the eyes and will not be subject to the influence of an atmosphere of strain. They should also learn the principles of central fixation in order that they may teach them to their children.

21

Treatment in Schools: Methods That Failed

No phase of ophthalmology, not even the problem of accommodation, has been the subject of so much investigation and discussion as the cause and prevention of myopia. Since hypermetropia was supposed to be due to a congenital deformation of the eyeball, and until fairly recently astigmatism was also supposed to be congenital in most cases, these conditions were not thought to call for any explanation or to admit of any prevention; but myopia appeared to be acquired. It therefore presented a problem of immense practical importance to which many eminent men devoted years of labour.

Voluminous statistics were collected regarding its occurrence, and they are still being collected. The subject has produced libraries of literature. But very little light is to be gained from the perusal of this material, and for the most part it leaves the reader with an impression of a hopeless confusion. It is impossible even to arrive at any conclusion as to the prevalence of the complaints, for not only has there been no uniformity of standards and methods, but none of the investigators has taken into account the fact that the refraction of the eye is not a constant condition but one which continually varies.

There is no doubt, however, that most children when they begin school are free from this defect, and that both the number of cases and the degree of the myopia steadily increase as the educational process progresses. Professor Hermann Cohn, whose report of his study of the eyes of more than ten thousand children in Germany first called general attention to this subject, found scarcely one per cent in the *Realschulen*, thirty to thirty-five in the gymnasia, and fifty-three to sixty-four in the professional schools. His investigations were repeated in many cities of Europe and America, and his observations, with some difference in percentages, were confirmed everywhere.

These conditions were unanimously attributed to the excessive use of the eyes for near work, though according to the theory that the lens is the agent of accommodation, it was a little difficult to see just why near work should have this effect. On the supposition that accommodation was effected by an elongation of the eyeball, it would have been easy to understand why an excessive amount of accommodation should produce a permanent elongation. But why should an abnormal demand on the accommodative power of the lens produce a change, not in the shape of that body but in the shape of the eyeball? Numerous answers to this question were proposed, but no one succeeded in finding a satisfactory one.

In the case of children it has been assumed by many authorities that, since the coats of the eye are softer in youth than in later years, they are unable to withstand a supposed intraocular tension produced by near work. When other errors of refraction, such as hypermetropia and astigmatism, believed to be congenital, were present, it has been supposed that the accommodative

167

struggle for distinct vision produced irritation and strain which encouraged the production of shortsightedness. When the condition developed in adults, the explanations had to be modified to fit the case, and the fact that a considerable number of cases were observed among peasants and others who did not use their eyes for near work led some authorities to divide anomaly into two classes, one caused by near work and one unrelated to it, the latter being conveniently attributed to hereditary tendencies.

As it was impossible to abandon the educational system, attempts were made to minimize the supposed evil effects of the reading, writing, and other near work which it demanded. Careful and detailed rules were laid down by various authorities as to the size of type to be used in schoolbooks, the length of the lines, their distance apart, the distance at which the book should be held, the amount and arrangement of the light, the construction of the desk, the length of time the eyes might be used without a change of focus, and so on. Even face-rests were devised to hold the eyes at the prescribed distance from the desk and to prevent stooping, which was supposed to cause congestion of the eyeball and thus encourage elongation. The Germans, with characteristic thoroughness, actually used these instruments of torture, Cohn never allowing his own children to write without one, 'even when sitting at the best possible desk'.

The results of these preventive measures were disappointing. Some observers reported a slight decrease in the percentage of myopia in schools in which the prescribed reforms had been made, but on the whole the injurious effects of the educational process were not eliminated to any extent.

Further study of the subject has only added to its difficulty, while at the same time it has tended to relieve the schools of much of the responsibility formerly attributed to them for the production of myopia. As the *American Encyclopedia of Ophthalmology* points out, 'the theory that myopia is due to close work aggravated by town life and badly lighted rooms is gradually giving ground before statistics.'

In an investigation in London, for instance, in which the schools were carefully selected to reveal any differences that might arise from the various hygienic, social, and racial influences to which the children were subjected, the proportion of myopia in the best-lighted building of the group was actually found to be higher than in the one where the lighting conditions were worse, although the higher degrees of myopia were more numerous in the latter than in the former.

It has also been found that there is just as much myopia in schools where little near work is done as in those in which the demand upon the accommodative power of the eye is greater. It is only a minority of children, moreover, that become myopic, yet all are subject to practically the same influences, and even in the same child one eye may become myopic while the other remains normal. On the theory that shortsightedness results from any external influence to which the eye is exposed, it is impossible to account for the fact that under the same conditions of life the eyes of different individuals and the two eyes of the same individual behave differently.

Because of the difficulty of reconciling these facts on the basis of the earlier theories, there is a disposition to attribute myopia to hereditary tendencies. But no satisfactory evidence on this point has been brought forward, and the fact that primitive peoples who have always had good eyesight become myopic just as quickly as any others when subjected to the conditions of civilized life, like the Indian pupils at Carlisle Institute, seems to be conclusive evidence against the suggestion.

The prevalence of myopia, the unsatisfactoriness of all explanations of its origin, and the futility of all methods of prevention, have led some writers of repute to the conclusion that the elongated eyeball is a natural physiological adaptation to the needs of civilization. Against this view two unanswerable arguments can be brought. One is that the myopic eye does not see as well as the normal eye even at the near-point; the other is that the defect tends to progression with very serious results, often ending in blindness.

If Nature has attempted to adapt the eye to civilized conditions by an elongation of the globe, she has done it in a very clumsy manner. It is true that many authorities assume the existence of two kinds of myopia: one physiological, or at least harmless, and the other pathological; but since it is impossible to say with certainty whether a given case is going to progress or not, this distinction, even if it were correct, would be more important theoretically than practically.

Into this slough of despair and contradiction the misdirected labours of a hundred years have led us. But in the light of truth the problem turns out to be a very simple one. In view of the facts given in Chapter 6, it is easy to understand why all previous attempts to prevent myopia have failed. All these attempts have aimed at lessening the strain of near work upon the eye, leaving the strain to see distant objects unaffected and totally ignoring the mental strain which underlies the optical one.

There are many differences between the conditions to which the children of primitive man were subjected and those under which the children of civilized races spend their developing years, besides the mere fact that the latter learn things out of books and write things on paper and the former did not. In the process of education, civilized children are shut up for hours every day within four walls, in the charge of teachers who are sometimes nervous and irritable. They are even compelled to remain for long periods in the same position. The things they are required to learn may be presented so that they are excessively uninteresting; and they are under a continual compulsion to think of the gaining of marks and prizes rather than the acquisition of knowledge for its own sake.

Some children endure these unnatural conditions better than others. Many cannot stand the strain, and thus schools become the hotbed not only of myopia but of all other errors of refraction.

22

Treatment in Schools: A Method That Succeeded

To repeat a very important principle: you cannot see anything with perfect sight unless you have seen it before. When the eye looks at an unfamiliar object it always strains more or less to see that object, and an error of refraction is always produced. When children look at unfamiliar writing or figures on the blackboard, distant maps, diagrams, or pictures, the retinoscope always shows that they are myopic, though their vision may be absolutely normal under other circumstances. The same thing happens when adults look at unfamiliar distant objects. When the eye regards a familiar object, however, the effect is quite different. Not only can it be regarded without strain, but the strain of looking at unfamiliar objects later is lessened.

These facts furnish us with a means of overcoming the mental strain to which children are subjected by the modern educational system. It is impossible to see anything perfectly when the mind is under a strain, and if children become able to relax when looking at familiar objects, they become able, sometimes in an incredibly brief space of time, to maintain their relaxation when looking at unfamiliar objects.

I discovered this fact while examining the eyes of

several hundred schoolchildren at Grand Forks, North Dakota. In many cases, children who could not read all of the letters on a test card in the first test read them in the second or third test. After a class had been examined, the children who had failed would sometimes ask for a second test, and then it often happened that they would read the whole card with normal vision. So frequent were these occurrences that there was no escaping the conclusion that in some way the vision was improved by reading the test card.

In one class I found a boy who at first appeared to be very myopic, but who, after a little encouragement, read all the letters on the test card. The teacher asked me about this boy's vision, because she had found him very nearsighted. When I said that his vision was normal she was incredulous, and suggested that he might have learned the letters by heart or been prompted by another pupil. He was unable to read the writing or figures on the blackboard, she said, or see the maps, charts and diagrams on the walls, and he did not recognize people across the street. She asked me to test his sight again, which I did, very carefully, under her supervision, the sources of error which she had suggested being eliminated. Again the boy read all the letters on the card. Then the teacher wrote some words and figures on the blackboard and asked him to read them. He did so correctly. Then she wrote additional words and figures, which he read just as well. Finally, she asked him to tell the hour by the clock, twenty-five feet away, which he did correctly.

Three other cases in the class were similar; their vision, which had previously been very defective for distant objects, became normal in the few moments devoted to testing their eyes.

It is not surprising that after such a demonstration the teacher asked to have a test card placed permanently in the room. The children were directed to read the smallest letters they could see from their seats at least once every day, with both eyes together and with each eye separately, the unused one being covered with the palm of the hand in such a way as to avoid pressure on the eyeball. Those whose vision was defective were encouraged to read the test card more frequently—but they needed no encouragement after they found that the practice helped them to see the blackboard and stopped the headaches and other discomforts previously resulting from the use of their eyes.

In another class of forty children, all between six and eight, thirty of the pupils gained normal vision while their eyes were being tested. The remainder did likewise later, under the supervision of the teacher, by means of exercises in distant vision with a test card. This teacher had noted every year for fifteen years that the opening of school in the fall all the children could see the writing on the blackboard from their seats, but before school closed the following spring all of them without exception complained that they could not see it at a distance of more than ten feet. After learning of the benefits to be derived from the daily practice of distant vision with familiar objects as the point of fixation, this teacher kept a test card in her classroom and directed the children to read it every day. The result was that for eight years no more of the children under her care acquired defective eyesight.

The teacher of this class had attributed the invariable deterioration in the eyesight of her charges during the school year to the fact that her classroom was in the basement and the light was poor. But teachers with

174

well-lighted classrooms had the same experience, and after the test card was introduced into both the well-lighted and the poorly lighted rooms, and the children read it every day, the deterioration of their eyesight ceased and, in addition, the vision of all improved. Vision which had been below normal improved, in most cases, to normal, while children who already had normal sight, usually reckoned at 20/20, became able to read 20/15 or 20/10. And not only was myopia eliminated, but the vision for near objects was improved.

At the request of the superintendent of schools in Grand Forks at that time, the system was introduced into all the schools of the city and was used continuously for eight years. During this time it reduced myopia among the children, which I found at first to be about six per cent, to less than one per cent.

A few years later the same system was introduced into some of the schools of New York City, with an attendance of about ten thousand children. Many of the teachers, however, neglected to use the cards, being unable to believe that such a simple method, and one so entirely at variance with previous teaching on the subject, could accomplish the desired results. Others kept the cards in a closet except when they were needed for the daily eye drill, lest the children should memorize them. Thus they not only put an unnecessary burden upon themselves but also did what they could to defeat the purpose of the system, which is to give the children daily exercise in distant vision with a familiar object.

A considerable number of teachers, on the other hand, used the system intelligently and persistently, and in less than a year were able to present reports showing that of three thousand children with imperfect sight, over one thousand had obtained normal vision by its means.

Some of these children, as in the case of children of Grand Forks, were relieved in a few minutes. Many of the teachers also were relieved, some of them very quickly. Sometimes the results of the system were nothing short of astonishing—but in the end the board of education and the eyeglass specialists couldn't agree, and gradually the use of test cards for this purpose was dropped.

In a class of mental defectives, where the teacher had kept records of the eyesight of the children for several years, it had been found that vision grew steadily worse as each term advanced. As soon as the test card was introduced, however, they began to improve. Then came a doctor from the local board of health who tested the eyes of the children and put glasses on all of them, even those whose sight was fairly good. The use of the card was then discontinued, as the teacher did not consider it proper to interfere while the children were wearing glasses prescribed by a physician.

Very soon, however, the children began to lose, break, or discard their glasses. Some said that the spectacles gave them headaches, or that they felt better without them. In the course of a month or so, most of the aids to vision which the board of health had supplied had disappeared. The teacher then felt herself at liberty to resume the use of the test card. Its benefits were immediate. The eyesight and the mental reactions of the children improved simultaneously, and soon many of them were drafted into the regular classes, because it was found that they were making as much progress in their studies as the other children were.

Another teacher reported an equally interesting experience. She had a class of children who did not fit into the other grades. Many of them were backward in their studies, some were persistent truants, and all of them had defective eyesight. A test card was hung in the classroom where all the children could see it, and the teacher carried out my instructions literally. At the end of six months all except two of the children had normal sight, and these two had definitely improved, while the worst incorrigible and the worst truant had become decent students.

To remove any doubts that might arise as to the cause of the improvement noted in the eyesight of the children, comparative tests were made with and without test cards. In one case six pupils with defective sight were examined daily for one week without the use of the card. No improvement took place. The card was then restored to its place and the group was instructed to read it every day. At the end of a week all had improved and five were completely normal. With another group of defectives the results were similar. During the week that the test card was not used, no improvement was noted; but after a week of excercises in distant vision with the card all showed marked improvement, and at the end of a month all were normal.

In order that there might be no question as to the reliability of the records of the teachers, in some cases the principals of the schools involved asked the board of health to send an inspector to test the vision of the pupils, and whenever this was done the records were found to be correct.

One day I visited the city of Rochester, New York, and while there I called on the superintendent of public schools and told him about my method of preventing myopia. He was very much interested and invited me to introduce it in one of his schools. I did so, and at the

177

end of three months a report was sent to me showing that the vision of all the children had improved, while quite a number of them had obtained normal vision in both eyes. The system, however, later met with the same end here that it had in New York City.

My method has been used in a number of other cities, and always the vision of all the children improved, many of them obtaining normal vision in the course of a few minutes, days, weeks, or months. It is difficult to prove a negative proposition, but since this method improved the vision of all the children who used it, it follows that none could have grown worse. It is therefore obvious that it must have prevented myopia. This cannot be said of any method of preventing myopia in schools which had previously been tried. All other methods are based on the idea that it is the excessive use of the eyes for near work that causes myopia, and all of them have admittedly failed.

It is also obvious that the method must have prevented other errors of refraction, a problem which previously had not even been seriously considered, because hypermetropia is supposed to be congenital and until not long ago astigmatism was also supposed to be congenital in the great majority of cases. Anyone who knows how to use a retinoscope, however, can demonstrate in a few minutes that both of these conditions are acquired; for no matter how astigmatic or hypermetropic an eye may be, its vision always becomes normal when it looks at a blank surface without trying to see. It may also be demonstrated that when children are learning to read, write, draw, sew, or do anything else that necessitates their looking at unfamiliar objects at the near-point, hypermetropia or hypermetropic astigmatism is always produced. The same is true of adults.

These facts strongly suggest that children need, first of all, eye education. They must be able to look at strange letters or objects at the near-point without strain before they can make much progress in their studies, and in every case in which the method has been tried it has been proved that this end is accomplished by daily exercise in distant vision with a test card. When their distant vision has been improved by this means, children invariably become able to use their eyes without strain at the near-point.

The method succeeded best when the teacher did not wear glasses. Not only do children imitate the visual habits of a teacher who wears glasses, but the nervous strain of which the defective sight is an expression produces in them a similar condition. In classes of the same grade, with the same lighting, the sight of children whose teachers did not wear glasses has always been found to be better than the sight of children whose teachers did wear them. In one case I tested the sight of children whose teacher wore glasses, and found it very imperfect. The teacher went out of the room on an errand, and after she had gone I tested them again. The results were very much better. When the teacher returned she asked about the sight of a particular boy, a very nervous child, and as I was proceeding to test him she stood before him and said, 'Now, when the doctor tells you to read the card, do it.' The boy couldn't see anything. Then she went behind him, and the effect was the same as if she had left the room. The boy read the whole card.

There are today in the schools of the United States several million children who have defective sight. This

179

condition prevents them from taking full advantage of the educational opportunities which the state provides, it undermines their health and wastes the taxpayers' money. If allowed to continue, it will be an expense and a handicap to these children throughout their lives. In many cases it will be a source of continual misery and suffering. And yet practically all of these cases could be relieved and the development of news one prevented by no more elaborate treatment than the daily reading of a test card.

Why should our children be compelled to suffer and wear glasses for want of this simple measure of relief? It costs almost nothing. In many cases, in fact, it would not be necessary even to purchase test cards, since they are already being used to test the eyes of the children. It places almost no additional burden upon the teachers and by improving the eyesight, health, disposition and mentality of their pupils, it greatly lightens their labours. No one would venture to suggest, further, that it could possibly do any harm.

Directions for Using a Test Card for the Improvement of Vision in Schools

The test card is placed permanently upon the wall of the classroom and every day children silently read the smallest letters they can see from their seats with each eye separately, the other being covered with the palm of the hand in such a way as to avoid pressure on the eyeball. This takes no appreciable amount of time and is enough to improve the sight of all children in one week and to eliminate all errors of refraction after some months, a year, or longer.

180

Children with markedly defective vision should be encouraged to read the card more frequently. Children wearing glasses should not be interfered with, as they are supposed to be under the care of a physician, and the practice will do them little or no good while the glasses are worn.

While not essential, it is a great advantage to have records made of the vision of each pupil at the time when the method is introduced, and thereafter at convenient intervals—annually or more frequently. This may be done by the teacher.

The records should include the name and age of the pupils, the vision of each eye tested at twenty feet, and the date. For example:

John Smith, ten, September 15, 19—
R. V. [vision of the right eye] 20/40
L. V. [vision of the left eye] 20/40
John Smith, eleven, January 1, 19—
R. V. 20/30
L. V. 20/15

A certain amount of supervision is absolutely necessary. At least once a year someone who understands the method should visit each classroom for the purpose of answering questions, encouraging the teachers to continue the use of the method, and making some kind of a report to the proper authorities. But it is not necessary that either the supervisor, the teachers, or the children understand anything about the physiology of the eye.

23

Mind and Vision

DEFECTIVE vision, as I have said, is the result of an abnormal condition of the mind. Glasses may sometimes neutralize the effect of this condition upon the eyes, and by making a person more comfortable may improve his mental faculties to some extent; but we do not alter fundamentally the condition of the mind, and by confirming it in a bad habit we may make it worse

It can easily be shown that among the faculties of the mind which are impaired when the vision is impaired is the memory; and as a large part of the educational process consists of storing the mind with facts, and as all the other mental processes depend upon one's knowledge of facts, it is easy to see how little is accomplished by merely putting glasses on a person who has 'trouble with his eyes'. The extraordinary memory of primitive people has been attributed to the fact that because of the absence of any convenient means of making written records they had to depend upon their memories, which were strengthened accordingly. But in view of the known facts about the relation of memory to eyesight it is more reasonable to suppose that the retentive memory of primitive man was due to the same cause as his keen vision, namely, a mind at rest.

The primitive memory, as well as the keenness of primitive vision, has been found among civilized people, and if the necessary tests had been made it would doubtless have been found that they always occur together, as they did in a case which recently came under my observation. The subject was a young girl with such marvellous eyesight that she could see the moons of Jupiter with the naked eye, a fact which was proved by her drawing a diagram of these satellites which exactly corresponded to the diagrams made by persons who had used a telescope.

Her memory was just as remarkable. She could recite the whole content of a book after reading it, as Lord Macaulay is said to have done, and she learned more Latin in a few days without a teacher than her sister, who had six diopters of myopia, had been able to do in several years. She remembered what she had eaten at a restaurant five years earlier, and she recalled the name of the waiter, the number of the building and the street on which it stood. She also remembered what she wore on this occasion and what everyone else in the party wore. The same was true of every other event which had awakened her interest in any way, and it was a favourite amusement in her family to ask her what the menu had been and what people had worn on particular occasions.

When the sight of two persons is different, it has been found that their memories differ in exactly the same degree. Two sisters, one of whom had ordinarily good vision, indicated by the formula 20/20, while the other had 20/10, found that the time it took them to learn eight verses of a poem varied in almost exactly the same ratio as their sight. The one whose vision was 20/10 learned eight verses of the poem in fifteen minutes, and the one whose vision was only 20/20 required thirty-one minutes to do the same thing.

After palming, the sister with ordinary vision learned eight more verses in twenty-one minutes, while the one with 20/10 was able to reduce her time by only two minutes, a variation clearly within the limits of error. In other words, the mind of the latter was already in a normal or nearly normal condition and she could not improve it appreciably by palming, but the former, whose mind was under a strain, was able to gain relaxation by palming and hence improve her memory.

Even when the difference in sight is between the two eyes of the same person, it can be demonstrated, as was pointed out in Chapter 10, that there is a corresponding difference in the memory, according to whether both eyes are open or the better eye closed.

The memory cannot be forced any more than the vision can be forced. We remember without effort, just as we see without effort, and the harder we try to remember or see, the less we are able to do so.

The things we remember are the things that interest us, and the reason we have difficulty in learning certain subjects is that we are bored by them. When we are bored our eyesight becomes impaired, boredom being a condition of mental strain in which it is impossible for the eye to function normally.

The youngster with the keen eyes, mentioned early in the chapter, could recite whole books if she happened to be interested in them. But she disliked mathematics and anatomy extremely, and not only could not learn them but became myopic when they were presented to her mind. She could read letters a quarter of an inch high at twenty feet in a poor light, but when asked to read numbers one to two inches high in a good light at ten feet she miscalled half of them. When asked to name the sum of two and three, she said four before finally deciding on five, and all the time she was occupied with this disagreeable subject the retinoscope showed that she was myopic. When I asked her to look into my eye with the ophthalmoscope she could see nothing, although a much lower degree of visual acuity is required to note the details of the interior of the eye than to see the moons of Jupiter.

A shortsighted young woman, to take the opposite of this case, had a passion for mathematics and anatomy and excelled in those subjects. She learned to use the ophthalmoscope as easily as the farsighted girl had learned Latin. Almost immediately she saw the optic nerve and noted that the centre was whiter than the periphery. She saw the light-coloured lines, the arteries; and the darker ones, the veins; and she saw the light streaks on the blood vessels. Some specialists never become able to do this, and no one could do it without normal vision. Her vision, therefore, must have been temporarily normal when she did it. Her vision for figures, although not normal, was better than for letters.

In both these cases the ability to learn and the ability to see went hand in hand with interest. One could read a photographic reduction of the Bible and recite verbatim what she had read, and could see the moons of Jupiter and draw a diagram of them afterwards. because she was interested in these things; but she could not see the interior of the eye, nor could she see figures even half as well as she saw letters, because these things bored her. But when it was suggested to her that it would be a good joke to surprise her teachers, who were always reproaching her for her backwardness in

185

mathematics, by making a high market in coming examination, her interest in the subject awakened and she contrived to learn enough to get a mark of 78. In the other's case, letters were antagonistic She was not interested in most of the subjects with which they dealt and therefore she was backward in those subjects and had become habitually myopic. But when she was asked to look at objects which aroused an intense interest, her vision became normal.

When one is not interested, in short, one's mind is not under control, and without mental control one can neither learn nor see. Not only the memory but all other mental faculties are improved when the eyesight becomes normal. It is a common experience with people cured of defective sight to find that their ability to do their work has improved.

A book-keeper nearly seventy years of age who had worn glasses for forty years found that after he had gained normal sight without glasses he could work more rapidly and accurately and with less fatigue than ever in his life before. During busy seasons, or when short of help, he worked for some weeks at a time from 7 A.M. until 11 P.M., and he insisted that he felt less tired at night after he was through than he did in the morning when he started. Previously, although he had done no more work than any other man in the office, it always tired him very much. He also noticed an improvement in his temper. Having been so long in the office, and knowing so much more about the business than his fellow employees, he was frequently appealed to for advice. These interruptions, before his sight became normal, were very annoying to him and often made him lose his temper. Afterwards, however, they caused him no irritation whatever.

In another case, symptoms of insanity were relieved when the vision became normal. A physician who had already been seen by many nerve and eye specialists came to me, not because he had any faith in my methods but because nothing else seemed to be left for him to do. He brought with him quite a collection of glasses prescribed by different men, and no two of them were alike. He told me that he had worn glasses for many months at a time without benefit, and then he had left them off and had been apparently no worse. Outdoor life had also failed to help him. On the advice of some prominent neurologists he had even given up his practice for a couple of years to spend the time on a ranch, but the vacation had done him no good.

I examined his eyes and found no organic defects and no error of refraction. Yet his vision with each eye was only three-fourths of the normal and he suffered from double vision and all sorts of unpleasant symptoms. He used to see people standing on their heads and little devils dancing on the tops of the high buildings. He also had other illusions too numerous to be mentioned here. At night his sight was so bad that he had difficulty in finding his way about, and when walking along a country road, he believed that he saw better when he turned his eyes far to one side and viewed the road with the side of the retina instead of with the centre. At variable intervals, without warning and without loss of consciousness, he had attacks of blindness. These caused him great uneasiness, for he was a surgeon with a large and lucrative practice and he feared that he might have an attack while operating.

His memory was very poor. He could not remember the colour of the eyes of any member of his family, although he had seen them all daily for years. Neither could he recall the colour of his house, the number of rooms on the different floors, or other details. The faces and names of patients and friends he recalled with difficulty or not at all.

This man's treatment proved to be very difficult, chiefly because he had an infinite number of erroneous ideas about physiological optics in general and his own case in particular. He insisted that all these should be discussed, and while the discussions were going on he received no benefit. Every day for hours at a time over a long period he talked and argued. His logic was wonderful, apparently unanswerable, and yet utterly wrong.

His eccentric fixation was of such high degree that when he looked at a point forty-five degress to one side of the big C on the test card he saw, the letter just as black as when he looked directly at it. The strain to do this was terrific and produced much astigmatism, but the patient was unconscious of it and could not be convinced that there was anything abnormal in the symptom. If he saw the letter at all, he argued, he must see it as black as it really was, because he was not colour blind. Finally he became able to look away from one of the smaller letters on the card and see it worse than when he looked directly at it. It took eight or nine months to accomplish this, but when it had been done the patient said that it seemed as if a great burden had been lifted from his mind. He experienced a wonderful feeling of rest and relaxation throughout his whole body.

When asked to remember black with his eyes closed and covered he said he could not do so, and he saw every colour but the black which one ought normally to see when the optic nerve is not subject to the stimulus of light. He had been an enthusiastic football player at

188

college, however, and at last he found that he could remember a black football. I asked him to imagine that this football had been thrown into the sea and that it was being carried outward by the tide, becoming constantly smaller but no less black. This he was able to do, and the strain floated with the football until, by the time the latter had been reduced to the size of a full stop in a newspaper, it was entirely gone. The relief continued as long as the patient remembered the black spot, but as he could not remember it all the time, I suggested another method of gaining permanent relief. This was to make his sight voluntarily worse, a plan against which he protested with considerable emphasis.

'Good heavens!' he said. 'Isn't my sight had enough without making it worse?,

After a week of argument, however, he consented to try the method, and the result was extremely satisfactory. After he had learned to see two or more lights where there was only one, by straining to see a point above the light while still trying to see the light as well as when looking directly at it, he became able to avoid the unconscious strain that had produced his double and multiple vision and was not troubled by these superfluous images any more. In a similar manner other illusions were prevented.

One of the last illusions to disappear was his belief that an effort was required to remember black. His logic on this point was overwhelming, but after many demonstrations he was convinced that no effort was required to let go, and when he realized this, both his vision and his mental condition immediately improved.

He finally became able to read 20/10 or more, and although more than fifty-five years of age, he also read diamond type at from six to twenty four inches. His night blindness was relieved, his attacks of day blindness ceased, and he told me the colour of the eyes of his wife and children. One day he said to me:

'Doctor, I think you for what you have done for my sight, but no words can express the gratitude I feel for what you have done for my mind.'

Some years later he called to tell me that there had been no relapse.

From all these facts it will be seen that the problems of vision are far more intimately associated with the mind than is ordinarily supposed, and that they can by no means be solved by putting concave, convex, or astigmatic lenses before the eyes.

24

The Fundamental Principles of Treatment

THE object of all the methods used in the treatment of imperfect sight without glasses is to secure rest or relaxation, first of the mind and then of the eyes. Rest always improves the vision. Effort always lowers it. Persons who wish to improve their vision should begin by proving these facts to themselves.

To demonstrate that strain lowers the vision, think of something disagreeable, some physical discomfort, or something seen imperfectly. When the eyes are opened, it will be found that the vision has been lowered. Also stare at one part of a letter on the test card, or try to see the whole letter all alike at one time This invariably lowers the vision, and may cause the letters to disappear. Another symptom of strain is a twitching of the eyelids which can be seen by an observer and felt by the patient with the fingers. This can usually be corrected if the period of rest is long enough. Many persons fail to secure a temporary improvement of vision by closing their eyes because they do not keep them closed long enough. Children will seldom do this unless a grown person stands by and encourages them. Many adults also require supervision.

The simplest way to rest the eyes is to close them for a longer or shorter period and think about something agreeable. This is always the first thing to do, and there are very few people who are not temporarily benefitted by it.

Palming

A still greater degree of rest can be obtained by closing and covering the eyes so as to exclude all the light. Close both eyes and cover them with the palms of both hands, the fingers crossed over upon the forehead. The mere exclusion of the impression of sight is often enough to produce a large measure of relaxation, although sometimes the strain is increased. As a rule, successful palming involves a knowledge of various other means of obtaining relaxation. The mere covering and closing of the eyes is useless unless at the same time mental rest is obtained. When you can palm perfectly you will see a field so black that it is impossible to remember, imagine, or see anything blacker, and when you are able to do this your sight will be normal.

Swinging

Demonstrate that swinging not only improves your vision but also relieves or cures pain, discomfort, and fatigue.

Stand with your feet about one foot apart, squarely facing one side of the room. Lift the left heel a short distance from the floor while turning the shoulders, head, and eyes to the right until the line of the shoulders is parallel with the wall. Now turn the body to the left, after placing the left heel upon the floor, and raise the right heel. Alternate looking from the right wall to the left wall, being careful to move the head and eyes with the movement of the shoulders. When swinging is practised easily, continuously, without effort and without paying any attention to moving objects, one soon realizes that it relaxes the tension of the muscles and nerves. (Remember, however, that the shorter you can eventually make the swing, the greater your improvement will be.)

Stationary objects move with varying degrees of rapidity. Objects located almost directly in front of you appear to move with express-train speed, and should be very much blurred. It is very important to make no attempt to see clearly objects which seem to be moving very rapidly.

Swinging seems to help especially people who suffer from eyestrain during sleep. Practising it fifty times or more just before retiring and just after rising in the morning has often prevented or relieved eyestrain during sleep.

Memory

When the sight is normal the mind is always perfectly at rest, and when the memory is perfect the mind is also at rest. Therefore it is possible to improve the sight by the use of the memory. Anything you find agreeable to remember is a rest to the mind, but for purposes of practice a small black object, such as a full stop or a letter of fine print, is usually most convenient. The most favourable condition for the exercise of the memory is, usually, with the eyes closed and covered, but by practice it becomes possible to remember just as well with the eyes open.

When you are able, with your eyes closed and covered, to remember perfectly a letter of fine print, it appears, just as it would if you were looking at it with the bodily eyes, to have a slight movement, while the openings in it appear whiter than the rest of the background. If you are not able to remember it, then shift consciously from one side of the letter to another and consciously imagine the opening whiter than the rest of the background. When you do this, the letter usually appears to move in a direction contrary to that of the imagined movement of the eye, and you are able to remember it indefinitely.

The reading every day of small familiar letters at the greatest distance at which they can be seen is a rest to the eyes, since the eye is always relaxed to some degree by looking at familiar objects.

Imagination

Imagination is closely allied to memory, for we can imagine only as well as we remember, and in the treatment of imperfect sight the two can scarcely be separated. Vision is largely a matter of imagination and memory. And since both imagination and memory are impossible without perfect relaxation, the cultivation of these faculties not only improves the interpretation of the pictures on the retina but improves the pictures themselves. When you imagine that you see a letter on the test card you actually do see it, because it is impossible to relax and imagine the letter perfectly and at the same time strain and see it imperfectly.

The following method of using the imagination has produced quick results in many cases. Look at the largest letter on the test card at the near-point, and you will usually be able to observe that a small area, about an inch square, appears blacker than the rest, and that when the part of the letter seen worst is covered, part of the exposed area seems blacker than the remainder. When the part seen worst is again covered, the area of maximum blackness is still further reduced. When the part seen best has been reduced to about the size of a letter on the bottom line, imagine that such a letter occupies this area and is blacker than the rest of the letter. Then look at a letter on the bottom line and imagine that it is blacker than the largest letter. If you can do this, you will at once become able to see the letters on the bottom line.

Flashing or Blinking

Since it is effort that spoils the sight, many persons with imperfect sight are able, after a period of rest, to look at an object for a fraction of a second. If the eyes are closed before the habit of strain reasserts itself, permanent relaxation is sometimes very quickly obtained. This practice I have called 'flashing' or 'blinking', and many persons are helped by it who are unable to improve their sight by other means. Rest the eyes for a few minutes by closing them or palming, and then regard for a fraction of a second a letter on the testcard, or a letter of fine print if the trouble is with near vision. Close the eyes immediately and repeat the process.

Central Fixation

When the vision is normal the eye sees one part of everything it looks at best and every other part worse in proportion as it is removed from the point of maximum vision. When the vision is imperfect it is invariably found that the eye is trying to see a considerable part of its field of vision equally well at one time. This is a great strain upon the eye and mind, as anyone whose sight is approximately normal can demonstrate by trying to see an appreciable area all alike at one time. At the near-point the attempt to see an area even a quarter of an inch in diameter in this way will produce discomfort and pain. Anything which rests the eye tends to restore the normal power of central fixation. It can also be regained by conscious practice, and this is sometimes the quickest and easiest way to improve the sight.

When you become conscious of seeing one part of your field of vision better than the rest, it usually becomes possible to reduce the area seen best. If you look from the bottom to the top of the big C on a test card and see the part not directly regarded worse than the part fixed, you may become able to do the same with the next line of letters, and thus you may become able to go down the card until you can look from the top to the bottom of the letters on the bottom line and see the part not directly regarded worse. In that case you will be able to read the letters.

Since small objects cannot be seen without central fixation, the reading of fine print, when it can be done, is one of the best of visual exercises, and the dimmer the light in which it can be read, and the closer to the eye it can be held the better it is for you.

196

Sunlight is as necessary to normal eyes as is rest and relaxation. If it is possible, start the day by exposing the closed eyes to the sun. Just a few minutes at a time will help. Get accustomed to the strong light of the sun by letting it shine on your closed eyelids. It is good to move the head slightly from side to side while doing this, in order to prevent straining. When you have become used to the strong light, raise the upper lid of one eye and look downward as the sun shines on the sclera. Blink when the desire to comes, or when you lose the power of relaxation. One cannot get too much sun treatment.

How to Practise with the Test Card

(1) Place the card permanently on the wall in a good light.

(2) Place yourself from ten to twenty feet from the card and read as far as you can without effort or strain. Over each line of letters are small figures indicating distance. Over the big C at the top is the figure 200. The big C, therefore, should be read at a distance of two hundred feet if the vision is normal.

(3) Now let us say you can only read as far as the fifth line at the distance indicated. Notice that the last letter on that line is an R. Now palm your eyes and remember the R. If you will remember that the left side is straight, the right side partly curved, and the bottom open, you will get a good mental picture of the R with your eyes closed. This mental picture will help you to see the letter directly underneath the R, which is a T. Use the same method at whichever line

197

the vision seems to fail: notice the last letter of the last line you can read, palm, get a good mental picture of the last letter seen, and you will find it easier to see the one directly beneath it.

(4) Now if you stare at the final letter, you will notice all the letters on that line begin to blur. It is beneficial to close your eyes quickly after you see the final letter, open them and shift to the first figure on that line. Then close your eyes and remember the first figure. You will become able to read all the letters on that line by closing your eyes for each letter.

It takes only a minute to rest the sight with the card. If you spend five minutes in the morning practising with the card, it will be a great help during the day. Also keep a record of each test in order to note your progress from day to day. Record the vision in the form of a fraction, with the distance at which the letter is read as the numerator and the distance at which it ought to be read as the denominator. For example, 20/20 is normal, 10/20 less than normal, and 25/20 better than normal.

Health Care in Orient Paperbacks

Dear Reader,

Welcome to the world of **Orient Paperbacks**—India's largest selling paperbacks in English. We hope you have enjoyed reading this book and would want to know more about **Orient Paperbacks.**

There are more than 400 **Orient Paperbacks** on a variety of subjects to entertain and inform you. The list of authors published in **Orient Paperbacks** includes, amongst others, distinguished and well-known names as Dr. S. Radhakrishnan, R.K. Narayan, Raja Rao, Manohar Malgonkar, Khushwant Singh, Anita Desai, Kamala Das, Dr. O.P. Jaggi, Norman Vincent Peale, Sasthi Brata and Dr. Promilla Kapur. **Orient Paperbacks** truly represent the best of Indian writing in English today.

We would be happy to keep you continuously informed of the new titles and programmes of **Orient Paperbacks** through our monthly newsletter, **Orient Literary Review.** Send in your name and full address to us today. We will start sending you **Orient Literary Review** completely free of cost.

Available at all bookshops or by VPP

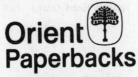

Orient
Paperbacks

Madarsa Rd, Kashmere Gate
Delhi-110 006, India